DYNAMIC DIET

Revealed: The Secret Superfoods That Help You Live Longer and Look Younger...

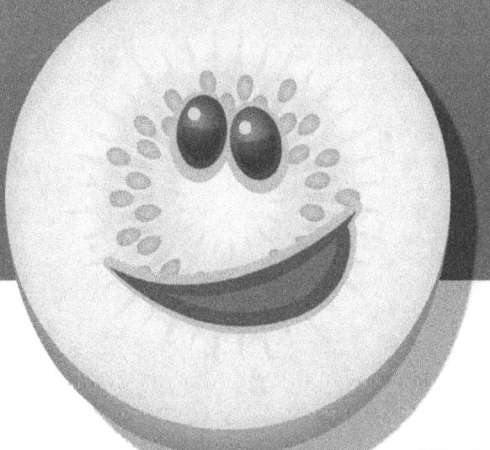

Elaine Hodgkinson

Dynamic Diet

Elaine Hodgkinson

About 'Dynamic Diet'

Published In the United Kingdom by Hodgkinson Publishing Limited
© Copyright Hodgkinson Publishing Ltd 2010 All Rights Reserved

Online: HodgkinsonPublishing.com

Super Food Listings:

- *Acai Berry*
- *Chinese Wolf Berry*
- *Pomegranate Fruit*
- *Oranges*
- *Goji Berry*
- *Spinach*
- *Broccoli*
- *Salmon*
- *Olive Oil*
- *Kiwis*
- *Green Tea*
- *Pepper*
- *Garlic*
- *Rosemary*
- *Ginger*
- *Basil*
- *Thyme*
- *Oregano*
- *Cinnamon*
- *Mint*
- *Licorice*
- *Bilberry*
- *Milk Thistle*
- *Echinacea*
- *Ginseng*
- *St. John's Wort*
- *Astragalus*
- *Ginko*
- *Flax*
- *Spirulina*
- *Boswellia*

Introduction

Most people in the world today are understandably anxious to improve the quality of their diets, but in today's fast food oriented world, this is easier said than done. It can be quite a challenge to eat healthy with so many unhealthy choices stocking the supermarket shelves and the menus of restaurants.

When improving your diet, however, it is important to be persistent, and to learn as much as you can about how diet can affect health. Many have long suspected that a good diet plays a vital role in good health, but many recent studies have shown that a good, balanced and healthy diet is much more important than even the experts ever suspected.

Creating an everyday diet that is both healthy and easy to follow is one of the single most important things anyone can do to improve their overall health and well-being. A good diet can improve not only the way we feel but the way we look as well. Many who follow a healthy diet rich in the best foods are able to look far younger than their actual age, and this healthy aging is but one of the many benefits of a healthy diet.

Many in the world of medicine, science and nutrition have long understood the value of good nutrition to good health. It would be virtually impossible to enjoy a healthy lifestyle over the long term without focusing on the foods you put into your body. Eating a healthy and balanced diet is one of the simplest, yet also most effective, changes you can make to help ensure a healthy body and a healthy future.

However, the benefits of a healthy diet go much further than simply feeling better, losing weight and gaining a higher degree of fitness. While things like weight loss and higher energy level are certainly worthy goals, proper nutrition can lead to a longer life, and many foods even have the ability to prevent many common diseases, including such killers as heart disease, stroke and even cancer.

While many foods provide vital nutrients, vitamins and minerals, there are a number of important foods whose benefits go far beyond simple nutrition. These so-called superfoods are valuable at preventing a number of diseases and they should form the basis of any disease prevention regimen.

From their role in preventing cancer to their role in reducing the effects of environmental pollutants, these superfoods are extremely valuable to a healthy lifestyle. This publication focuses on 30 of the most valuable superfoods available to you in some form or another. These are foods that can help you live longer, feel better and enjoy a healthier lifestyle and greater level of fitness.

Some of these superfoods have been known to science for centuries or even millennia, while others are more recent discoveries. What they all have in common, however, is their ability to prevent disease. These superfoods are among the most nutrient dense on the market, and most of them are both widely available and inexpensive. Whether they are included in the diet as herbs, whole foods or supplements, their role In a balanced diet simply cannot be overstated.

While many foods have made the superfood claim over the years, the list of actual bona fide superfoods is much shorter. The top nutrient dense foods generally acknowledged to have the characteristics of superfoods are:

- Acai Berry
- Astragalus
- Basil
- Bilberry
- Boswellia
- Broccoli
- Chinese wolf berry
- Cinnamon
- Echinacea
- Flax (flax seed oil)
- Garlic
- Ginger
- Ginko
- Ginseng
- Goji berry
- Green tea

- Kiwis
- Licorice
- Milk thistle
- Mint
- Olive oil
- Oranges
- Oregano
- Pepper
- Pomegranate fruit
- Rosemary
- Salmon
- Spinach
- Spirulina
- St. John's Wort
- Thyme

These superfoods are quite different from one another, but they all have one thing in common, and that is that they are the most nutrient dense, organically active foods on the market.

Many of these foods have the ability to boost the function of the immune system while others provide the phyto-nutrients and antioxidants needed to ward off common diseases, while still others combine a number of other benefits to provide the biggest bang for your nutritional buck.

These foods are available in a number of different forms, from delicious edible varieties, to wonderful herbs used in cooking to excellent supplements. Many of these superfoods come in more than one form, making it easy to add variety to your life while enjoying a healthier lifestyle and longer life.

Acai Berry

Classification: Edible, supplement

Origin: For many years, the Acai berry has been a well-kept secret of the Amazon rainforest. The rainforests of the Amazon are thought to hold the key to treating many ailments and common diseases, and for thousands of years the indigenous peoples of the Amazon region have known about the many health-enhancing benefits of the Acai berry.

The Acai berry grows wild on top of many palm trees that are native to the rainforests of Brazil and the Amazon basin. Local farmers in the area harvest the fruit of the tree, and it is used to make a healthful fruit pulp. This fruit pulp is then quickly frozen in order to preserve its nutrient value.

The Acai berry itself is a deep purple color, and it is quite rich in a number of important nutrients, including many of the most valuable antioxidant vitamins.

Major benefits of the acai berry: The Acai berry is thought to have a significant impact on heart health, and on the health of the cardiovascular system. In particular, the Acai berry contains a very high concentration of compounds known as anthocyanins. These compounds are the same ones thought to be responsible for giving red wine its widely reported health benefits.

In addition to these anthocyanins, Acai berries are known to contain large amounts of protein and fiber, as well as both omega-6 and omega-9 fatty acids. These omega fatty acids have been studied for years as a way to protect the heart from damage, and they may be able to reduce the amount of cholesterol in the blood, thereby providing possible protection from heart attacks, strokes and other common cardiovascular complications.

These anthocyanins are known to have significant health benefits, and they are the subjects of many studies. Many people are looking for ways to capture the many health benefits that have been associated with the consumption of red wine, but without the calories and other negative consequences of red wine consumption. The rich, delicious fruit of the acai berry may be able to provide these important health benefits.

Perhaps the most important health benefit of the acai berry, however, is its strong impact on the aging process. As a matter of fact, the acai berry is generally acknowledged to be one of the top superfoods for anti-aging. The antioxidant benefits of the acai berry, combined with the fatty acids it contains, make this one of the most important superfoods on the market.

The acai berry is thought to have an antioxidant content which is a full 10 times greater than that found in grapes, and twice as high as those found in blueberries. As a matter of fact, the acai berry is widely acknowledged to have the highest nutritional value of any fruit in the world, and this has earned it the acai berry the title of superfood.

Additional information: For such a tiny fruit, the Acai berry seems to have a great many heart healthy benefits, and the secret that has been part of Amazon culture for thousands of years is slowly spreading to the rest of the world. The Acai berry is a rich source of antioxidant vitamins, protein, fiber and heart protecting fatty acids, and it has an important role to play in protecting our good health.

Acai berries can be purchased whole and eaten as part of a healthy diet, but they are most often encountered in juice form. Acai berry juice is widely available both in health food stores and from many Internet retailers. As with other kinds of juice, it is important to ensure that the Acai berry juice you buy is made with 100% pure juice, and that it contains no artificial ingredients or added sugar.

As the popularity of the Acai berry continues to grow, and as its value to good health continues to get out, it is likely that this little purple fruit will become more widely available. In coming years, Acai berries are likely to be available at traditional grocery stores and supermarkets in addition to health food stores and Internet retailers.

When choosing between products made with the Acai berry, it is important to choose only the highest quality products, and to look for products that have been frozen quickly after harvest. How the Acai berries are handled after harvest can have a significant impact on their health benefits, so it is important to buy your Acai berry juice from those who use the best manufacturing methods.

Chinese Wolfberry

Classification: Edible

Origin: As its name implies, the Chinese wolfberry is native to China and other parts of Asia, and it has long been part of traditional Oriental medicine. The health benefits of the Chinese wolfberry were known as far back as 1000 A.C., and the traditional Chinese Medica reference book contains many references to this important superfood.

The Chinese wolfberry grows wild on bushes, mainly in the northwest region of China. The wolfberry has been grown and cultivated for thousands of years, both for its good taste and its nutritional and medicinal value. The Chinese wolfberry blooms from April through October and it is harvested from June to October depending on local growing conditions.

Major benefits of the Chinese wolfberry: The Chinese wolfberry is thought to have the important ability to strengthen the organs of the body, particularly the eyes, kidneys and liver. The Chinese wolfberry is well known to the world of herbal medicine, and it is included in many traditional herbal formulas.

Health benefits of the Chinese wolfberry include treating such conditions as insomnia, fatigue, dizziness, vision problems, ringing in the ears and headaches. The Chinese wolfberry is also thought to be effective at treating such serious conditions as tuberculosis, chronic liver disease, high blood pressure and diabetes.

Chinese wolfberry is also thought to be of great value in maintaining and boosting the health of the immune system, keeping the liver healthy and improving eyesight. In addition, wolfberry is thought to be effective in maintaining healthy levels of blood pressure and blood sugar.

The Chinese wolfberry has long been known to be of value to human health, and it has been used in Chinese medicine for thousands of years. The fruits of the wolfberry are used in many traditional herbal formulas, and they are still used in such formulas today. In addition, the fruits of the wolfberry are delicious and extremely nutritious, and this bright red fruit is increasingly making its way into both supermarkets and health food stores.

The fruits of the Chinese wolfberry have been used for a number of chronic health problems, especially those involving tired legs, dizziness, headaches, insomnia and chronic liver diseases. In addition, wolfberry, both used as a food and a nutritional supplement has shown great promise at treating high blood pressure, tuberculosis and diabetes as well.

Additional information: The fruit of the Chinese wolfberry can be prepared in a number of ways. The fruit is often chewed and eaten, much as one would eat raisins. In addition, Chinese wolfberry can be used in a number of teas, soups and stews. There is even a Chinese wolfberry wine that is common in Oriental cultures. The fruits of the Chinese wolfberry are oblong in shape and very juicy. This juice, and the wolfberry itself, both have a very sweet taste.

The primary ingredient in the Chinese wolf berry, the one thought to be responsible for the many benefits of this superfood, is known as Lycium Barbarum Polysaccharide

(LBP).   The amount of LBP contained in wolfberries will vary according to the type of berry and the growing conditions, with the top quality wolfberries being those which contain the highest concentration of LBP.

Pomegranate fruit

Classification: Edible

Origin: The pomegranate fruit is common throughout the countries of the Middle East, in Iran and in India, and the pomegranate has long played a role not only in the cuisine but also in the medicine of those traditional cultures.

The pomegranate fruit has long been used in traditional folk medicine, and it has played a major role in the medicine of many indigenous cultures. Some of the many ailments that pomegranates have been used to treat include sore throats, rheumatism and inflammation. In addition to its many health benefits the pomegranate provides a delicate, tangy and sweet flavor.

Major benefits of the pomegranate fruit: Some recent studies of pomegranate fruit and pomegranate juice has suggested that this fruit contains almost three times as many antioxidants as are found in red wine and green tea. In addition to these benefits, pomegranate fruit contains significant amounts of potassium, niacin and vitamin C, as well as plenty of fiber.

In traditional medicine, the pomegranate fruit has long been used to treat such conditions as sore throats, rheumatism and general inflammation. It is thought that the strong antioxidant content, and the quality of those antioxidants, is able to boost the immune system and have a significant effect on overall health and well-being.

In addition, pomegranates are being studied for their possible role as an anticancer food. The antioxidant content of the pomegranate fruit, in addition to its concentration of other vitamins and minerals, are thought to play a protective role in preventing many types of cancer.

The strong antioxidant content of pomegranates make them among the most popular and most delicious of all superfoods. Whether you choose to eat fresh pomegranates or enjoy a delicious glass of pomegranate juice, these fruits are a delicious way to improve your diet.

Additional information: The pomegranate fruit has a tough rind that can be brownish or dark red, and the fruit is similar in size to an apple or orange. It is the juicy red pulp that is the edible part of the fruit.

From ancient times on, the pomegranate fruit has been linked to fertility, and the pomegranate is featured prominently in the mythology of ancient Egypt and Greece.

When choosing pomegranate fruits, it is important to choose those with the richest color, and those that feel heavy for their size. Dry looking or wrinkled pomegranate fruits are best left at the store. In the refrigerator pomegranate fruits will keep for up to three months, while their unrefrigerated shelf life is reduced to two or three days. In most parts of the United States, fresh pomegranate fruits are available in September, October and November.

In addition to fresh pomegranate fruit, the juice of the pomegranate is another great way to enjoy this popular superfood. Pomegranate juice can be drunk on its own, or used to make a variety of delicious foods, such as jellies, sauces and marinades. In addition, pomegranate seeds can be sprinkled over salads and desserts, and also used as a garnish for meats, poultry and fish dishes.

Oranges

Classification: Edible

Origin: Orange trees grow in tropical locations around the world but they are best known in the southern and western parts of the United States. In the U.S., oranges are big business in Florida and California, as well as in Georgia and other southern states.

Major benefits of oranges in the diet: Oranges and other foods rich in antioxidant vitamins are being studied for their possible usefulness in preventing cancer and other diseases. In addition to their high content of healthful vitamin C, oranges contain more than 170 phytochemicals, including more than 20 compounds in the carotenoid family. These carotenoids have shown incredible promise at fighting many kinds of cancer, and oranges are the best single source of many of these compounds.

In addition to these carotenoids, oranges also contain important compounds called limonoids. It is these limonoids that give oranges and other citrus fruits their tangy flavor, and these compounds are thought to be strong anticancer agents. Oranges are among the richest sources of limonoids.

And of course the best-known benefit of oranges is its strong content of vitamin C. Vitamin C, in addition to its strong antioxidant properties and possible role in fighting cancer, has been studied for everything from treating colds and flu to helping cuts heal more quickly.

Oranges are perhaps the richest sources of vitamin C available, and the average sized orange contains an amazing 92% of the vitamin C needed in the daily diet. Vitamin C is the most prevalent water-soluble antioxidant vitamin in the body, and it has been shown to reduce the cell damage associated with aging and environmental pollution.

Additional information: As rich sources of vitamin C, phytonutrients and many other important vitamins, oranges are among the most important foods in the supermarket. In addition to being nutritious, oranges are delicious and inexpensive as well. It is no wonder oranges are being increasingly recognized as one of the most valuable superfoods.

Oranges are perhaps the best known of all superfoods. Just about everyone has enjoyed a delicious orange, and a glass of fresh 100% orange juice is one of the best and healthiest ways to start any day. A glass of orange juice with breakfast can get your day off to a great start while helping improve your health.

When choosing to drink orange juice, however, it is important to choose only those juices that are made with 100% real juice. Choosing juices with lower fruit content, or juices with added sugar or artificial ingredients, could reduce and possibly even eliminate the awesome power of this superfood.

Goji berry

Classification: Edible

Origin: The goji berry is native to the Himalayans, and it grows well in this harsh environment. The natives of the Himalayan region were among the first to discover the important health benefits of this important food. The goji berry has long enjoyed an honored place in the world of Oriental medicine, and it has been used throughout the Asian world for thousands of years. The modern world is just now beginning to discover the important benefits of the goji berry.

Major benefits of the goji berry: The goji berry may be the most important anti-aging food available today. The power of this superfood lies largely in its ability to reduce the effects of aging. This tiny red fruit is thought to have a significant impact on many degenerative and aging related ailments.

The goji berry contains important compounds known as polysaccharides, known also as phytonutrient compounds. These compounds are thought to play an important role in the way the cells of the body carry out instructions and communicate with one another. Scientists often refer to these polysaccharides as master molecules, because of their ability to control many elements of the body and the immune system.

Perhaps the easiest and most effective way to enjoy the many benefits of the goji berry is by including one of the many goji juices on the market as part of your daily diet. Goji juice can provide many important health benefits, including all six essential amino acids and the 21 important trace minerals that make up the content of the goji berry.

As with any type of juice, it is important that the goji juice you buy contains only 100% pure juice, and that it be free of any artificial ingredients or added sugar. It is important not to negate the important benefits of the goji berry by adding unhealthy ingredients such as sugar or artificial preservatives.

Additional information: It is important to know that the goji berries grown in their traditional home in the valleys of the Himalayas contain a greatest concentration and better balance of polysaccharides than those grown elsewhere in the world, so the origin of the goji berries or supplements you buy is an important consideration.

The goji berry can be enjoyed in a variety of ways, from eating the fruits themselves to taking a daily supplement that contains this valuable fruit. In addition to goji berries, goji juice is widely available in a variety of supermarkets, natural food retailers and health food stores. When shopping for goji juice, it is important to choose those made with 100% real juice, and to avoid those with added sugar or artificial ingredients.

Spinach

Classification: Edible

Origin: Spinach is believed to have originated in ancient Persia, the country that is now known as Iran. Spinach was introduced to China sometime in the seventh century when it was presented to China as a gift from the king of Nepal.

In Europe, spinach has a much shorter history than many other popular vegetables. Spinach was first introduced to Europe sometime in the 11th century, when the Moors introduced it into Spain. As a matter of fact for some time the English referred to spinach as the Spanish vegetable.

Spinach grows quite well in most temperate climates, and the Netherlands and United States are among the biggest commercial growers of spinach on the market today.

Major benefits of eating spinach: There are many reasons to enjoy the dark green leafy vegetable known as spinach. For many years spinach has been touted as a health food, and this superfood certainly lives up to its reputation. Spinach is a rich source of many important vitamins and minerals, including vitamin C, iron, calcium and beta-carotene.

Spinach is also a rich source of dietary fiber, thought to play an important role in protecting the body from many forms of cancer. As a matter of fact, the compounds contained in spinach are being studied for their possible role in preventing many forms of cancer, including such major killers as lung cancer. One reason may be the high concentration of vitamin K found in spinach. Vitamin K has long been associated with cancer prevention, and spinach is one of the very best sources of this vital nutrient.

This possible role as a cancer preventative is only one of the healthful effects of spinach. In addition, spinach may also play an important role in protecting the heart and cardiovascular system from damage. Spinach should be a part of every diet, but it may be even more important to those at risk for heart disease and stroke.

Spinach has also shown real promise at preventing cataracts. Some studies have suggested that this eye protection is due to the high concentration of beta-carotene found in spinach. Beta-carotene is thought to play an important role in eye health, and this may mean that the consumption of spinach can help protect the eyes from cataracts and other common vision problems.

One other reason for the eye protecting benefits associated with spinach may be its high concentration of lutein and zeaxanthin. These important carotenoids, similar to beta-carotene, are not only strong antioxidant vitamins, but they are thought to help protect against cataracts as well.

Spinach in the diet is also thought to help control high levels of homocysteine in the bloodstream. Recent studies have shown that a diet high in vitamin C, folic acid, beta-carotene and other nutrients found in spinach had lower homocysteine levels in their blood.

Additional information: The vitamins contained in spinach are also thought to play a role in preventing macular degeneration and other aging related diseases of the eye. Macular degeneration is the most common eye diseases in the elderly, and spinach and other dark green leafy vegetables are thought to help protect the body from these degenerative conditions.

In addition to its value as a superfood, spinach is low in price, widely available, and useful in a great number of recipes. Spinach is delicious and nutritious, and there is no reason not to include it in a healthy diet.

When choosing spinach it is important to choose spinach with a vibrant color and leaves of the richest and darkest green. It is important to avoid spinach that shows signs of yellowing. The leaves of spinach should appear fresh and tender, and they should not be bruised or wilted. In addition, it is important to avoid spinach that has a slimy coating on it, as this can be a sign of decay.

Fresh spinach should be loosely packaged in a plastic bag, and it should be stored in the crisper in the refrigerator. Spinach kept in the crisper drawer of the refrigerator will keep for up to four days, but it is important to use it as quickly as possible to ensure both freshness and good taste.

Spinach should not be washed prior to storage, since the excess moisture could cause it to spoil prematurely. Cooked spinach does not keep well and should not be stored. While spinach can be frozen after it has been blanched for two minutes, frozen spinach will develop a very soft texture. For this reason frozen spinach should not be allowed to completely thaw before being cooked.

Broccoli

Classification: Edible

Origin: It is thought that broccoli was first cultivated in Italy, back in the times when Rome ruled the world. Broccoli was first developed from wild cabbage, a plant that looks more similar to collard greens than to modern broccoli. The popularity of broccoli quickly spread throughout the entire Near East, and it was appreciated for its edible flower heads. This led broccoli to be further cultivated in Italy. Broccoli was introduced to the United States back in colonial times, where it was introduced by the many Italian immigrants who came to the new world.

Since it was first cultivated, broccoli has been a popular vegetable, renowned for its easy preparation, its health benefits and its great taste. For many years broccoli has been a favorite with health conscious consumers. In most parts of the country broccoli is available year round, but its traditional season runs from October through May, and broccoli bought at this time of year is generally the most flavorful and the most nutritious.

Broccoli is actually a member of the cabbage family and it is closely related to cauliflower, which is also closely resembles. The Italian word for broccoli, broccoli, translates to "cabbage sprout" for its appearance. Broccoli provides a number of different tastes and textures, from the soft florets to the crunchy and fibrous stems and stalks.

Major benefits of eating broccoli: Broccoli provides a number of important benefits, but perhaps the most important of these benefits is possible protection against many forms of cancer. Broccoli contains phytochemicals such as sulforaphane and indoles, which provide strong anticancer benefits. In particular, research into indole-3-carbinol has shown that this compound may help to inhibit chemicals that promote the growth of tumors, thereby providing protection against cancers and tumor formation.

The various compounds contained in broccoli have also been shown to help prevent cancer cells from spreading to other parts of the body and to boost the effects of various detoxifying enzymes.

In addition to its role in fighting cancer, broccoli may be able to improve the appearance of the skin as well. That is because sulforaphane, one of the major compounds found in broccoli and similar vegetables may be able to boost the detoxifying effects of liver and skin cells. Some recent studies have also suggested that the compounds found in broccoli may be able to repair the sun damage to the skin.

The compounds found in broccoli are also thought to provide extensive benefits to the heart and cardiovascular system. Many recent studies have suggested that the nutrients and other compounds present in broccoli may be able to prevent the heart from damage, due to the high level of flavonoids and other antioxidant vitamins it contains.

Broccoli is thought to provide these important effects through the presence of antioxidant vitamins, which have the ability to disarm the free radicals that are part of the normal aging process. These free radicals can damage the cells of the body, leading to premature aging and other harmful effects. Antioxidant vitamins, like those found in broccoli, are thought to have the ability to mitigate the cell damage done by these free radicals.

In addition, broccoli may have significant effects at preventing cataracts and other degenerative diseases of the eye. That is because broccoli contains such powerful phytochemical vitamins in the carotenoid family as lutein and zeaxanthin. Both of these phytochemicals are present in high concentrations in the lens of the eye. In a recent study those who consumed broccoli every day were found to have a lower incidence of cataracts and other eye diseases than those who did not consume broccoli on a regular basis.

Broccoli is also a strong source of calcium, and it is therefore important to keeping the bones healthy and preventing osteoporosis. As a matter of fact, other than milk and other dairy products, broccoli is one of the very richest sources of calcium on the market. And broccoli provides all these bone healthy benefits without the fat and excess calories found in milk, ice cream and other dairy products.

Broccoli may have important abilities at preventing ulcers as well, since broccoli has been shown to be effective against the helicobacter pylori bacterium thought to be responsible for most peptic ulcers.

In addition to these other important benefits, the compounds in broccoli are thought to be effective at boosting the immune system. The many vitamins and minerals contained in broccoli can have a strong effect on the immune system, therefore helping to prevent many common diseases and aging related ailments.

Broccoli is also a rich source of folic acid, a vitamin that is crucial to preventing many of the most common birth defects. Therefore, women of childbearing age are strongly advised to eat plenty of broccoli. The folic acid in broccoli and other foods helps to protect the fetus from common birth defects, but the time to get that folic acid is before you get pregnant. By the time a woman knows she is pregnant, the harmful effects of insufficient folic acid may have already occurred.

Additional information: In addition to these important benefits, broccoli may also be effective at preventing rheumatoid arthritis. High doses of the many vitamins and other nutrients present in broccoli have been shown to be effective at preventing the effects of rheumatoid arthritis in many clinical trials.

When choosing broccoli it is important to select those heads with the richest, darkest color, as this broccoli will have both the best flavor and the best nutrient value. It is also important to choose broccoli heads whose floret clusters are of compact size and which are not bruised. The stems and stalks of the broccoli should be firm but tender, and no slimy spots should be evident, either on the stems or the florets. Any leaves attached to the broccoli head should have a vibrant color and not be wilted.

Fresh broccoli is quite perishable, and it is important to use it as quickly as possible after purchase. Broccoli should be stored in the crisper drawer of the refrigerator, and it will keep this way for up to four days. Broccoli should not be washed prior to storage, since excess water will reduce its shelf life.

Broccoli that has been blanched can be frozen and will stay good for up to a year. Any cooked broccoli should be placed into a tightly covered dish or container and stored in the refrigerator. Leftover cooked broccoli will only keep for a day or two in the refrigerator so it is important to use it up as quickly as possible.

Salmon

Classification: Edible

Origin: For as many years as there have been people, there have been people who enjoyed the healthful benefits and great taste of salmon. From the countries of Scandinavia and Russia to the United States and Europe, salmon is both a tasty treat and a staple of the diet.

While salmon are found swimming in many parts of the world, much of the commercially produced salmon today comes from the cold waters of the Pacific Northwest, eastern Canada, Norway, Greenland and Alaska.

Salmon contains a nutrient density found in few other foods, including the omega-3 fatty acids known to protect the heart from damage and lower cholesterol levels.

Major benefits of eating salmon: Eating salmon has many health benefits, but perhaps the most important benefit of salmon is its ability to protect the heart and cardiovascular system. That is because salmon contains all-important omega-3 fatty acids, and it is these fatty acids that have been shown to provide important heart protecting benefits.

In addition, the omega-3 fatty acids contained in salmon have been shown to improve the ratio of good cholesterol to bad cholesterol and to lower the overall levels of cholesterol and triglycerides in the blood as well.

The heart healthy benefits of salmon have long been known, and the evidence that salmon protects the heart from heart disease, stroke and high cholesterol has been growing with every passing year. Many recent studies have shown that salmon has the ability to protect the heart and cardiovascular system, through the presence of omega-3 fatty acids and other important nutrients.

In particular, eating salmon and other fish rich in omega-3 fatty acids have been shown to provide the following important benefits:

> Lowering the cholesterol and triglycerides in the bloodstream
> Improving the ratio of good cholesterol to bad cholesterol
> Helping to prevent the formation of blood clots
> Helping to inhibit the thickening of arteries
> Preventing obesity and improving insulin response in diabetics

Eating salmon may also provide important protection against stroke, and many studies have shown that the nutrients in salmon can help to prevent strokes, both by lowering the total cholesterol in the blood and helping to reduce the formation of the blood clots that can lead to stroke.

The heart healthy benefits of salmon are not limited to reducing the incidence of stroke and heart disease, however. Regular consumption of salmon has also been shown to help prevent arrhythmias of the heart. This protection was most evident when eating boiled or baked fish, while fried fish provided no such protection.

One of the omega-3 fatty acids found in salmon has also been shown to be effective at reducing inflammation. This fatty acid, known as EPA, is thought to provide anti-inflammatory effects by producing resolvins. These resolvins, which the body makes from EPA, are thought to improve blood flow to the joints, thereby reducing the inflammation associated with a number of ailments.

Salmon may even have the ability to protect the skin against sun damage, and perhaps even provide protection against skin cancer. It is thought that the consumption of omega-3 fatty acids, such as those found in salmon, may help to protect the skin from the damage associated with excess sun exposure, including perhaps skin cancer.

And of course salmon and other fish have long been thought of as brain food, and for good reason. There is strong evidence to suggest that eating salmon on a regular basis may protect the brain as well as the body from the degenerative effects of aging.

In addition to general brain protection and memory enhancement, salmon may provide protection against serious diseases like Alzheimer's. Eating salmon and other cold-water fish has been shown to be associated with a significantly lower risk of developing Alzheimer's disease. It is thought that these protective benefits are also a result of the omega-3 fatty acids that are contained in salmon and similar fish.

Regular consumption of salmon has also been associated with a substantial reduction in the risk of a number of cancers, including ovarian and various digestive tract cancers. It is thought that the nutrients in salmon provide protection against the cell breakdown associated with the formation of cancer tumors, and cancer prevention is one more important reason to eat salmon as often as possible.

In addition to ovarian cancer, regular salmon consumption has been associated with lower levels of such killers as pancreatic cancer, and with lower levels of stomach, mouth, colon, rectal and esophageal cancer as well.

The reason for this cancer protection seems to lie not only in the high concentration of omega-3 fatty acids contained in salmon, but in the fact that salmon is a strong source of selenium as well. Selenium is known to be very important to good health, and it is important to the proper function of many metabolic pathways, including those involved in immune system function and thyroid metabolism.

Additional information: The health benefits of fish have been well known for many years, and salmon is one of the most beneficial of all fish. This cold-water fish has a number of important health benefits, and there is no reason not to include regular servings of salmon in your diet.

Salmon is available in a great many different forms, including whole salmon, salmon steaks and salmon fillets. In addition, salmon is available in canned, frozen, smoked and dried varieties.

Whenever possible, it is important to choose wild salmon over its farm raised competition. There are worries that farm raised salmon could pose a cancer risk due to the accumulated PCBs and other environmental pollutants to can accumulated in the fat of farm-raised salmon. While the health benefits of eating salmon greatly outweigh its risks, eating wild salmon provides all the benefits of this superfood without introducing any unnecessary risks.

Olive oil

Classification: Edible

Origin: Olives are one of the oldest foods known to man, and the history of olive oil is nearly as old. Olives are thought to have originated on the island of Crete between five and seven thousand years ago. Since the most ancient times, olive trees were used to provide food, fuel and timber, and many civilizations saw olives as symbols of peace and wisdom. Olive oil has been a part of the human diet for at least five thousand years, and it continues to be an important element of good health in today's world as well.

Olives and olive oil were brought to what is now the United States as far back as the 15th and 16th century, brought by Portuguese and Spanish explorers. The Franciscan missionaries introduced olives and olive oil to California during the late 18th century.

Olive oil has long been a staple of cooking in many Mediterranean countries, and it is a rich part of the Mediterranean diet, which has been associated with a reduced risk of heart disease and other common health problems. Much of the cultivation of olives for olive oil still takes place in these Mediterranean countries, with Spain, Italy, Greece, Portugal and Turkey being important producers of olives and olive oil.

Olive oil is one of the most versatile of all the superfoods, and it is equally at home with pasta, fish, meat and salads. In addition, olive oil is available throughout the year at an excellent price.

Major benefits of eating olive oil: Olive oil is one of the most delicious, and also one of the healthiest of all oils used in cooking. Unlike many less healthy oils, olive oil is polyunsaturated oil, and it is rich in menstruated fat, which researchers have discovered has many health benefits. Olive oil is also one of the richest sources of vitamin E, one of the most important antioxidant vitamins in the diet.

This strong antioxidant content may be responsible for the fact that olive oil has been associated with protection against many chronic degenerative diseases and aging related ailments. Consumption of olive oil is thought to provide protection against such conditions as atherosclerosis, asthma, diabetes, arthritis and colon cancer. In addition, olive oil is thought to provide protective benefits against the effects of a high fat diet.

Olive oil is also thought to have many heart healthy benefits. Studies have revealed that those whose diets are rich in olive oil are less at risk of arthrosclerosis. Studies have suggested that that the fats contained in olive oil are less likely to become oxidized and thereby harm the heart than the fats contained in other kinds of oil.

In addition to its other effects on the heart and cardiovascular system, olive oil is also thought to provide protection against high blood pressure, and some studies have suggested that olive oil may even have the ability to reduce high blood pressure in those who suffer from the condition.

It is thought that olive oil may contain a number of anticancer benefits as well, and many studies into the cancer fighting effects of olive oil are underway. In particular, many of these studies have focused on the ability of olive oil to prevent breast cancer from forming.

Better control of blood sugar is another important benefit of olive oil, as is better control of inflammation. The anti-inflammatory and blood sugar regulating properties have long been known, and these properties are the subject of further study.

Additional information: In addition to its many health benefits, olive oil is versatile, delicious and easy to use. It is thought that simply replacing other less healthy cooking oils with healthier olive oil can have a significant impact on health and well being.

There are many ways to work olive oil into the daily diet, from dressing up a salad with olive oil and balsamic vinegar to sprinkling olive oil over vegetables or pasta salad. Olive oil is an important part of any healthy diet.

In addition, substituting olive oil for other types of oil in the diet can have a significant impact on body weight. Many studies have shown that this small change can lead to a healthier diet and a healthier weight. There is no doubt that olive oil is one of the healthiest of all cooking oils, and it is important to incorporate this healthy oil into all your cooking.

For many cooks, nothing beats the taste sensation and health benefits of making their own olive oil from scratch. Many gourmet stores sell olive presses, and these can be a great way to make your own olive oil for healthy cooking.

While most olives are still sold in cans and jars, a number of whole food retailers are beginning to make them available in large bulk barrels. These bulk barrels can provide cooks with a great way to experiment with the many different varieties of olives on the market, so if your local food retailer offers fresh olives they are definitely worth a look.

Kiwis

Classification: Edible

Origin: The kiwi fruit is native to China, and kiwis were known to the Chinese as Yang Tao. The kiwi fruit was first introduced to New Zealand from China by missionaries early in the 20th century and the first commercial plantings of kiwi took place several decades later. Kiwi fruits are also known as Chinese gooseberries, reflecting their Oriental origins.

Kiwi fruits were first introduced to American restaurants in 1961, and an American produce distributor helped to introduce them to the supermarkets and grocery stores of the country. Today, kiwi fruits are available in most supermarkets and grocery stores around the country, and it is loved for its nutritional value, its unique appearance and its great taste.

Today, much of the commercial production of kiwi fruit takes place in Italy, New Zealand, France, Japan, Chile and the United States, and this fuzzy coated fruit continues to be popular with many people.

Major benefits of kiwi fruit: Kiwi fruit is rich in many vital phytonutrients, as well as containing a great many important vitamins and minerals that are important to good health.

One of the most significant health benefits of kiwi fruits is their ability to protect DNA. This DNA protecting effect is thought to play a strong role in the prevention of cancer and other diseases, as well as promoting overall good health. Kiwi fruit is known to contain a number of important nutrients, including vitamin C and beta-carotene. In addition, kiwi contains a number of other flavonoids and carotenoids which have been shown to provide strong antioxidant activity. It is thought that these phytonutrients may be responsible for the ability of kiwi fruit to protect DNA.

Kiwi fruit is among the most nutrient dense of all fruits and this delicious superfood contains many of the most important fat-soluble antioxidant vitamins, including vitamin E and vitamin A. Kiwi fruit contains vitamin A in the form of beta-carotene, and allows kiwis to provide strong protection against the cell damage that can be caused by free radicals in the body.

In addition to protecting the DNA and the health of cells, kiwi fruit is thought to help protect the colon as well. Part of the reason for the colon protection provided by kiwi fruit is the fact that kiwis are a rich source of dietary fiber. It is thought that dietary fiber has the ability to reduce cholesterol in the blood, and that it may even play a role in reducing the risk of colon cancer.

In addition, the high concentration of vitamin A contained in kiwi fruit suggests that it may play an important role in protecting people against macular degeneration. Macular degeneration is the most common eye disease among the elderly, and vitamin A is known to play a role in reducing the risk of this serious degenerative eye disease. In addition to vitamin A, it is thought that other nutrients contained in kiwi fruit, such as beta-carotene, vitamin C and vitamin E, may provide vital eye protection and help to guard against macular degeneration and other common vision problems.

Kiwi fruit may even provide the same type of heart protection that aspirin does. As a matter of fact, enjoying a few kiwi fruit every day can significantly reduce the amount of triglycerides in the blood and lower the risk for blood clots. This makes kiwi fruit a great alternative to the blood thinning protection provided by aspirin, without the side effects that aspirin and other anti-inflammatory medications can provide.

Additional information: To properly choose kiwi fruits, gently apply pressure to the fruit while holding it between the thumb and forefinger. Those kiwi fruits with the sweetest taste will yield to this gentle pressure. Kiwi fruits that are too soft, shriveled or bruised should be avoided, as should those that have damp spots.

Those kiwi fruits that do not yield to gentle pressure are not yet ripe, and they have not yet reached the peak of their sweetness. These kiwi fruits can be left to ripen for a few days to a week at room temperature. Care should be used to avoid exposure to sunlight or excessive heat while the fruits are ripening. Once ripe, kiwi fruits can be stored either in or out of the refrigerator.

It is important not to store kiwi fruits near other fruits and vegetables, as the ethylene gas emitted by those fruits and vegetables can quickly cause the kiwi fruits to become overripe.

Green Tea

Classification: Culinary herbs

<u>Origin</u>: Green tea, like black tea and oolong tea, is derived from the tea plant and it is thought to have originated in the area of the world that now encompasses western China, northern India and the country of Tibet.

Chinese legend holds that tea was discovered by the emperor Shen-Nung in the year 2737 B.C. The story holds that the leaves from a wild tea bush accidentally fell in a pot of water the emperor was boiling, and a new drink was born. No matter what its provenance, tea is the most popular drink in the world, and green tea in particular is thought to have many important health benefits.

Tea has been mentioned in literature and recorded history for thousands of years, with the earliest mention of tea thought to have occurred in the year 59 B.C. By the year 780 A.D., marked by the publication of a book by Lu Yu called The Classic of Tea, the cultivation and brewing of tea was considered a fine art.

The tradition of India holds that tea was discovered by the Buddhist monk known as Siddhartha sometime in the sixth century. The legend holds that Siddhartha, a former prince turned monk, traveled north from India to China, vowing to meditate without sleeping for a period of nine years. After he reached Canton in the year 519 A.D., after meditating for five years, Siddhartha was overcome by overwhelming drowsiness. As if by divine inspiration, Siddhartha chewed the leaves of a nearby tree. After chewing these leaves, his drowsiness vanished and a feeling of alertness returned.

It was of course the tea tree that provided these remarkable effects, and allowed him to keep his vow of a nonstop nine-year meditation. The legend goes that Siddhartha carried these magical leaves with him as he continued his journey to the land of Japan. Other Buddhist monks quickly came to see the value of tea, and they used it to remain alert while meditating. These Buddhist monks used tea to create a simple drinking ritual that would be later formalized as the well-known Japanese tea ceremony.

From Japan, where tea was widely consumed by the ninth century, tea continued to spread its influence to the island of Java, the Dutch East Indies and many other corners of the world. By the 16th century, European traders coming to and from the Far East brought tea to the European continent, and by the 18th century, the influence of tea had spread across Europe, including of course England, where it remains the national drink to this day.

In the world today, it is not China but India that is the number one tea producer. Other major tea producing countries include Sri Lanka, Kenya, Indonesia, Turkey, Russia, Iran, the United States and Bangladesh.

Major benefits of green tea: There are many healthful drinks on the market, but few enjoy the strong reputation of the superfood known as green tea. For thousands of years the Chinese have known about the benefits of green tea, and this drink has been used to treat everything from headaches and depression to insomnia and digestive problems.

Green tea has shown significant promise at fighting many types of cancer. In one frequently cited study, there was a sixty percent decrease in the risk of esophageal cancer among those who drank green tea on a regular basis. The study found that a compound contained in green tea was able to inhibit the formation of cancerous cells.

In addition to its possible role as a cancer fighter, green tea is thought to have the ability to lower levels of both total cholesterol and bad (LDL) cholesterol. In addition, green tea has shown promise in reducing high blood pressure, preventing and treating rheumatoid arthritis and boosting the immune system.

The secret to the health effects of green tea are thought to lie in its high concentration of polyphenols. The most significant of these healthful compounds is thought to be epigallocatechin gallate (EGCG). EGCG has long been regarded as a strong antioxidant, and it has been shown to help kill cancer cells without injuring the healthy tissues of the body. EGCG is also thought to play a role in stopping the growth of cancer cells.

Green tea is also thought to be important to heart health, perhaps due to the ability of EGCG to lower cholesterol in the blood and reduce the formation of blood clots. That is why scientists are continuing to study green tea in relation to the so-called French paradox. Scientists and others have long been amazed by the fact that the French, who eat diets high in fat and other unhealthy elements, suffer from much lower levels of heart disease than Americans.

The answer to the French paradox may lie in the healthy benefits of red wine consumption, particularly in a compound known as resveratrol, which is thought to help reduce the effects of a fatty diet. The main ingredient in green tea is thought to be twice as powerful as a heart protector as the compounds found in red wine.

Green tea is also thought to have special benefits for those with high levels of triglycerides in the bloods. These harmful blood lipids are known to play a significant role In the development of heart disease, and there is considerable evidence that green tea can lower the levels of triglycerides in the blood.

It is thought that the mix of compounds found in green tea are able to inhibit the formation of pancreatic lipase, which as an enzyme secreted by the pancreas. This in turn has a strong effect on the rate at which these fats are broken down into triglycerides. Since the rise in triglycerides in the blood that often follows a meal is a risk factor in coronary artery disease, it is thought that following a fatty meal with one or two cups of green tea may have a protective effect on the heart and cardiovascular system.

Another important heart healthy benefit of green tea lies in its ability to prevent the formation of blood clots. The catechins in green tea help to thin the blood, thus helping to prevent blood clots from forming. In particular, green tea is thought to prevent inflammatory compounds found in fatty foods from forming.

While green tea is important in preventing heart disease, it may be even more important for those who have suffered a heart attack or who have heart disease to consume green tea. There is a great deal of research that has suggested that green tea may be able to help prevent further heart and cardiovascular damage in those who have suffered a previous heart attack. In addition, regular consumption of green tea has been shown to speed recovery following a heart attack or stroke.

The healthy compounds in green tea have been shown to minimize the death of heart cells following a heart attack or stroke, and the ECGC contained in green tea also appears to increase the recovery of those heart cells which have already been damaged, thus allowing the heart tissues to recover in a more timely manner and reducing possible damage to other organs.

The damage minimizing effects of green tea are not limited to the heart, however. The compounds contained in green tea have also been shown to be very protective of brain cells. It is thought that the brain cell protective functions of green tea work in much the same way as their heart protective functions and this suggests that green tea consumption may be able to help mitigate the damage which occurs following a stroke.

Green tea consumption has also been shown to have a strong impact on blood pressure, and the compounds in green tea have been shown to both help prevent high blood pressure and to lower high blood pressure in those who already suffer from it.

Green tea may even be able to prevent many forms of cancer, and these possible anticancer benefits are the subject of much ongoing research into the benefits of green tea. It is thought that the catechins contained in green tea, are able to interfere with the growth factors associated with cancer. These catechins appear to produce this effect by effectively shutting down the relay stations used by cancer to grow. These relay stations, known to science as tyrosine kinase receptors, are essential for a number of processes which turn normal cells into cancer cells, and it is thought that green tea may be able to prevent the development and growth of cancer by interfering with the growth factors cancer relies upon.

The anticancer benefits of green tea have continued to be documented in many studies, and the ability of green tea to prevent cancer has been continually documented. The evidence for the anticancer benefits of green tea has become so overwhelming that there are plans for developing the compounds found in green tea into cancer preventing and cancer fighting drugs.

Among the many cancers the compounds in green tea are thought to fight are such major cancers as prostate cancer, bladder cancer, ovarian cancer, breast cancer, childhood brain tumors, colon cancer, and lung cancer,

In addition it is thought that green tea may have the ability to improve the effectiveness of drugs used to treat cancer while lessening many of their unpleasant side effects. In particular, one of the active compounds in green tea, the amino acid known as theanine, has been shown to reduce the side effects of many chemotherapeutic agents while helping to increase their effectiveness.

Green tea is also being studied for its ability to improve the insulin sensitivity of type 2 diabetics. Many population studies have suggested that the compounds found in green tea may be able to prevent type-2 diabetes as well, in addition to improving the glucose tolerance and insulin sensitivity of those who have already developed type-2 diabetes.

In addition to these important benefits, green tea is being studied for its possible ability to fight the osteoporosis that all too often afflicts the elderly. Green tea is known to promote healthy bones and teeth by helping to protect the osteoblasts, which are responsible for building bones from the destructive effects of free radicals.

The compounds in green tea are also thought to play a protective role in the liver. Protecting the liver is essential to good health, since all impurities and pollutants taken into the body are filtered through the liver. It is thought that the antioxidants found in green tea are able to minimize the liver damage done by free radicals, and this may account for much of its protective benefits.

And of course dieters have long known about the fat loss benefits of green tea. Green tea is thought to have a simulative effect on the metabolism, and every dieter knows that a faster metabolism means a greater number of calories burned. In addition, the compounds found in green tea are thought to increase the effectiveness of exercise, helping people burn more calories with the same amount of exertion.

Green tea is thought to have a particularly profound effect on what is known as visceral fat. This special type of fat accumulates within the tissues that line the abdominal cavity and surround the intestines and internal organs. Visceral fat is thought to be more dangerous than fat deposits on the thighs and hips, so reducing this type of fat is generally acknowledged to have the most important health benefits.

Another important benefit of green tea for dieters is the fact that it is thought to increase exercise endurance. Many people who drink green tea on a regular basis report being able to exercise longer without becoming tired, and many athletes swear by the effects of green tea on endurance.

It is thought that the catechins contained in green tea are able to stimulate the usage of fatty acids by the cells of the muscles and the liver. This ability of muscle cells to burn more fat means a reduction of the speed at which glycogen is used up and this translates to the ability to exercise for longer lengths of time. This same effect on the ability of muscle cells to burn fatty acids is thought to be responsible for the weight loss effects of green tea consumption.

Pepper

Classification: Culinary herbs, edible

Origin: Pepper is derived naturally enough from the pepper plant. The pepper plant is actually a large woody vine that has been known to grow to heights of more than thirty feet. Pepper plants are common in the hot and humid climates found in the tropics of many countries.

The pepper plant vines begin to grow their traditional small white flowers at the age of three to four years, and it is those small white flowers that develop the berries more commonly known as peppercorns. These peppercorns are then ground to make the spice we know as pepper.

Major benefits of pepper: One of the most striking benefits of the superfood known as pepper seems to be its ability to aid the digestive system. Pepper is known to improve digestion and the health of the intestinal system as well. Digestive problems are among the most common complaints, and pepper seems to have a strong effect on improving the digestion of food.

For this reason pepper is thought to be important in preventing such common conditions as irritable bowel syndrome, diverticulitis and other common ailments of the digestive system.

Pepper is thought to provide this protective impact on the digestive system through the stimulation it provides to the taste buds. This stimulation of the taste buds in turn causes the stomach to increase its production of the hydrochloric acid that is so important to the proper digestion of the foods we eat. If sufficient quantities of hydrochloric acid are not present by the time the food reaches the stomach, such problems as heartburn, indigestion and other digestive problems may occur. By stimulating the taste buds, and therefore the production of stomach acid, pepper may help to avoid these common digestive issues.

In addition to its ability to prevent a number of other digestive problems, pepper is also able to reduce intestinal gas, thus providing a good solution to a common and embarrassing problem. The ability to reduce intestinal gas is also thought to be related to the increased production of hydrochloric acid in the stomach.

In addition, pepper is also known to have important antibacterial properties, and to contain significant levels of antioxidant vitamins as well. These antibacterial and antioxidant properties may mean pepper is able to fight common diseases, including perhaps even heart disease and cancer. With all these benefits going for it, there is no reason not to add a pinch of pepper to every meal you serve your family.

Additional information: In ages past, pepper was so valuable that it was even used as a form of currency, and pepper was often offered as a sacrifice to the gods worshipped by those ancient peoples. In today's world, however, pepper is plentiful, inexpensive, healthy and available year round.

Pepper can be purchased in a number of different varieties, including whole peppercorns and ground pepper. Some chefs swear by the nutritional and culinary benefits of grinding fresh peppercorns, while others prefer the convenience of fresh ground pepper. No matter what the form, however, pepper is one of the least expensive and most effective of all superfoods.

When using fresh ground pepper in recipes, it is best to buy the whole peppercorns and grind them using a pepper mill just prior to adding them to your favorite recipe. In addition to providing a superior flavor to your food, buying whole peppercorns will ensure that you get pure, unadulterated pepper. Commercially produced pepper is often mixed with other spices; grinding your own pepper will help ensure you are getting only the richest and most flavorful pepper.

If you do choose the convenience of ground pepper, it is important to ensure that the spice has not been irradiated, since irradiating pepper has been shown to decrease its content of vitamin C.

When storing ground pepper it is best to keep it in a tightly sealed glass container which is stored in a dark, cool and dry location. While ground pepper will remain fresh for up to three months, the shelf life of peppercorns is virtually endless.

Garlic

Classification: culinary herbs, edible

Origin: The herb known today as garlic is native to central Asia, and it is one of the longest cultivated plants in the entire world. Garlic has been cultivated for over 5000 years, with the residents of ancient Egypt widely believed to be the first to cultivate this herb.

Indeed, garlic played an important role in Egyptian culture. Not only was garlic endowed by the ancient Egyptians with sacred qualities and placed in tombs with other prized possessions, but it was also provided to the slaves who built the pyramids as a way to increase their physical endurance and strength. This ability to increase physical strength was also valued by the Romans and the Greeks, and their athletes were known to consume garlic prior to sporting events, while their soldiers often consumed garlic before heading off to war.

Garlic was brought to various parts of the world through the influence of migrating tribes and various explorers. By the sixth century B.C. the herb known as garlic was well known in both China and India. Indian healers in particular used the herb for its therapeutic qualities.

Throughout many thousands of years, garlic has been used both for its medicinal and its culinary values. The past few decades in particular, though, have seen a resurgence in the popularity of garlic for therapeutic purposes.

In the world today, the leading producers of garlic are the United States, Spain, India, China and South Korea, but the herb is cultivated and used throughout the world.

Major benefits of garlic: For many years garlic has been regarded as an incredibly powerful food, and garlic may well be the original superfood. Many modern scientific studies have backed up the anecdotal evidence that garlic provides many important health benefits. It is thought that the same compounds which give garlic its strong aroma and rich flavor are able to protect against many common health conditions.

It is thought that garlic may provide important protection against some types of cancer. Garlic is thought to provide this effect through its ability to neutralize certain cancer causing compounds and slowing the growth of tumors.

For many years the world of traditional medicine has regarded garlic as a wonder drug, and garlic has been traditionally been used to treat conditions ranging from the common cold to the Bubonic plague. While it may not be a cure for the plague, garlic is known to have great healing powers. When choosing garlic for its healing power, the stronger the odor of the garlic clove, the greater its medicinal value will be. This is because the sulfur compounds which give garlic its strong odor and rich flavor are the same ones responsible for its healing power.

Additional information: Many feel that organically grown garlic provides a higher sulfur content, and therefore a greater healing power, than non-organic varieties. In addition, others who want to reap the many health benefits of garlic without the unpleasant odor can turn to garlic capsules, tablets and other supplements.

Garlic, whether eaten as part of a healthy diet or as a supplement, has been shown to provide many strong health benefits. Garlic may provide antibiotic properties, and it has even shown usefulness as a mosquito repellent.

When adding raw garlic to the diet, it is important not to take too much too soon. Excessive consumption of garlic can produce unpleasant side effects such as irritation and damage to the digestive system. In addition, there are those who suffer allergies to garlic. While those allergies are rare, those who suffer garlic allergies may experience such symptoms as fever, headache and skin rashes.

It is also important to know that garlic acts as a blood thinner, so those scheduled for surgery should avoid garlic prior to any scheduled surgery. It is also important to keep your physician informed of all medications you are taking, including over the counter medications and supplements.

For superior flavor and nutrition, nothing can beat the power of fresh garlic. While garlic powders, garlic flakes and garlic paste may be more convenient, they are not as flavorful or as nutritious as fresh garlic.

When choosing fresh garlic it is important to choose cloves which are plump and on which the outside skin has not been broken. Garlic can be selected by gently squeezing the bulb between the fingers. The best garlic will feel firm to the touch and not be damp.

Garlic cloves which are shriveled, too soft or moldy are best left in the grocery store. The same goes for garlic cloves that have begun to sprout. All these things can be signs of decay, and this will cause the garlic to be of inferior flavor. Size is not generally an indication of quality with garlic, so it is best to choose the size clove according to how much your recipe calls for. Fortunately fresh garlic cloves are available in grocery stores and supermarkets all year round, so finding fresh garlic should not be much of a challenge.

Fresh garlic can be stored either loosely covered or uncovered in a cool dark place. It is important to keep the fresh garlic away from sunlight and other heat sources, as this will help to maintain its freshness. Garlic does not need to be refrigerated, and while it can be frozen, doing so will reduce the richness of its flavor and change its texture as well.

Rosemary

Classification: culinary herbs, edible

Origin: Although it is now grown throughout the temperate regions of Europe and the Americas, rosemary is actually native to the Mediterranean region. Rosemary has been prized as both a seasoning and as an herbal medicine for thousands of years.

For many years, rosemary was thought to help improve and strengthen memory, and it is still used for this purpose today. In ancient Greece, students studying for an exam would place a sprig of rosemary in their hair, and mourners at funeral services would throw rosemary into the grave as a symbol of their memories.

Major benefits of rosemary: Rosemary has traditionally been used as a memory enhancer, and it continues to be used to boost memory and brain function to this day. In addition, rosemary contains many compounds that are thought to be good at stimulating the immune system, improving digestive function and increasing circulation.

In addition, rosemary contains many compounds that have strong anti-inflammatory properties, a fact that may make rosemary useful in the treatment of asthma attacks. Rosemary has been shown effective at reducing the severity of asthma attacks, and this property of the herb remains the subject of much research.

Rosemary has also been shown to help improve blood flow to the brain, and to improve concentration. This effect of rosemary may be responsible for its traditional use as a memory enhancer.

Additional information: Rosemary is often grown in home herb gardens, and rosemary is in fact one of the easiest herbs to grow and use at home. Many cooks swear by the superior taste of fresh rosemary, and growing rosemary as a part of a home herb garden can be a great way to provide a steady and low cost supply of this delicious and nutritious herb.

In general, it is better to choose fresh rosemary instead of the dried variety. The flavor of fresh rosemary is far superior to that of the dried herb, and fresh rosemary will help your recipes turn out much better.

Sprigs of fresh rosemary should look vibrant and fresh and should have the color of sage green. Rosemary sprigs with dark spots or yellow spots should be avoided. Another excellent way to enjoy fresh rosemary year round is to grow it yourself in a home herb garden. Rosemary is easy to grow in an herb garden, and growing your own will ensure you have a steady supply of this delicious superfood.

For those who prefer the convenience of the dried herb, it is often better to buy it in a spice market or organic grocery store, as the quality to be found there is often superior to that which can be found in traditional supermarkets. It is also a good idea to look for organically grown rosemary whenever possible, as this will help ensure that the herbs are free of pesticide residue and that they have not been irradiated. Irradiating rosemary and other herbs has been shown to decrease the concentration of healthful carotenoids in the herb.

Fresh rosemary can be stored in the refrigerator, in either its original packaging or a dampened paper towel. In addition, fresh sprigs of rosemary can be stored in ice cube trays, either in water or in fresh stock. These rosemary infused ice cubes can come in handy when preparing fresh soups, stews and other meals.

Ginger

Classification: culinary herbs, edible

Origin: The herb known as ginger is native to Southeast Asia, and the various cuisines of Asian countries have long used ginger in their cooking. Ginger has long been featured in the writings of China, India and many Middle Eastern countries, and it has been prized for its medicinal and culinary qualities, as well as for its strong and vibrant aroma.

It is thought that the ancient Romans first imported this herb from china nearly two thousand years ago, and its popularity has continued to spread, until today it is used throughout the entire world. Today the top producers of ginger for the commercial market include India, Fiji, Jamaica, Indonesia and Australia.

Major benefits of ginger: Ginger has long been known for its healing properties as well as its good taste, and practitioners of Chinese, Japanese and Indian medicine have long known of its value.

One of the most significant benefits of ginger seems to be its ability to reduce nausea, and ginger is being studied as a possible way to avoid the nausea and vomiting often associated with chemotherapy treatment.

Ginger is also thought to have a profound effect on the circulation, and it is felt that it has an important role to play in reducing the incidence of heart disease. Scientists are not yet certain whether these benefits are derived from increased circulation or some other, as yet unknown, mechanism.

Another important benefit of ginger may be its ability to prevent and treat motion sickness, and many frequent travelers swear by the effectiveness of ginger for this purpose. Taking a small amount of ginger prior to travel has proven remarkably effective for many people.

In addition, the ant nausea effects of ginger may offer a natural way to treat the morning sickness and nausea that can accompany pregnancy. Ginger is currently being studied for its effectiveness as an anti morning sickness treatment, and many women swear by the power of ginger in the diet to reduce the uncomfortable effects of pregnancy.

In addition, ginger is thought to have strong anti-inflammatory effects, due to the presence of powerful anti-inflammatory compounds known as gingerols. The presence of these gingerols is thought to explain why so many of those who suffer from osteoarthritis and rheumatoid arthritis enjoy a reduction in their levels of pain as well as an increase in mobility when they eat ginger frequently.

In addition to these important benefits, ginger is even thought to play an important role in the prevention of colorectal cancer. Again the gingerols contained in this spice are thought to be responsible for its protective impact. These gingerols are the same compounds responsible for giving ginger its distinctive flavor and aroma, and these same compounds may be able to inhibit the growth of colorectal cancer cells. This anticancer benefit of ginger is the subject of much ongoing study, and it may be one of the most important roles of this superfood.

As with other valuable superfoods, ginger is also thought to provide a boost to the immune system. A strong and vibrant immune system is essential to good health, and ginger is thought to have the ability to boost the effectiveness of the immune system.

This may be one of the reasons that ginger has traditionally been used at the first sign of a cold or the first symptoms of the flu. It is thought that the warming and flushing action of ginger help to promote healthy sweating, which can be important to fighting off the effects of colds and flu. In addition, it is thought that the flushing and sweating associated with consumption of ginger may speed the detoxification process, thus providing a boost to the immune system and a shorter duration of colds, flu and other common infections.

Additional information: Most major grocery store chains and supermarkets carry fresh ginger root year round, and ginger is generally inexpensive as well as effective. When choosing ginger, it is important to look for the firmest roots, and those that have a strong aroma. The stronger the aroma, the more aromatic it will be when used in your recipes.

If at all possible, it is best to choose fresh ginger instead of the dried spice. Not only does fresh ginger provide a better flavor and pleasing aroma, but it also contains higher concentrations of the gingerols that are responsible for many of the health benefits of this superfood. In addition, fresh ginger contains higher levels of the protease that provides the anti-inflammatory benefits of ginger.

Fresh ginger root is easily found in the produce sections of many grocery stores and supermarkets. Good ginger root will be smooth, firm and mold free, and fresh ginger root is generally available in two different forms – young ginger root and mature ginger root. Mature ginger root is the most frequently seen variety, and it features a tough skin that must be peeled prior to use. In general young ginger is only available in Asian markets, and its skin does not require peeling.

Fresh ginger root can be stored for up to three weeks in the refrigerator as long as it has not yet been peeled. Unpeeled ginger root can be kept in the freezer for up to six months. Dried ginger powder must be kept in a dark, cool and dry place and should be stored in a tightly sealed container. It can also be stored in the refrigerator, where it can be kept for up to a year.

Basil

Classification: culinary herbs, edible

Origin: While basil is now grown throughout the world, it is native to India, Africa and Asia, and basil is widely used in a variety of world cuisines, including Thai cooking, Italian cuisine, Vietnamese culture and Laotian cuisine.

The name basil comes from an old Greek word "basilikohn", which translates to royal. This name origin reflects the attitude the ancient Greeks held toward basil, which was considered to be both noble and sacred. In India, basil was traditionally held as an icon of hospitality, while in Italy it was seen as a symbol of love.

Major benefits of basil: One of the things that makes basil such an important superfood is its value as a DNA protectant, as well as its antibacterial properties. In particular, basil contains a wide array of active compounds known as flavonoids. These compounds are thought to provide protection from disease at a cellular level. In studies of two of these flavonoids contained in basil – orientin and vicenin, they were found to protect cell structures and from radiation damage. This ability of the compounds in basil to protect cells and chromosomes could make it valuable in the fight against cancer, as well as a variety of degenerative diseases associated with aging.

In addition, the herb known as basil may be able to protect against excess growth of bacteria. These antibacterial properties of the herb are thought to be associated with its volatile oils, including linalool, estragole, cineole, sabinene, eugenol, limonene and myrcene. Studies in the laboratory have shown basil to be effective at reducing the growth of many different kinds of bacteria, including E. coli and listeria.

In addition to its usefulness as an herb, the essential oil obtained from the leaves have shown the capability of restricting the growth of many types of pathogens, including many which have evolved to be resistant to many antibiotics. This pathogen fighting ability is one of the most exciting and potentially valuable benefits of basil.

In addition to these specific benefits, basil is a rich source of many nutrients, including calcium, phosphorus, vitamin A and vitamin C. Basil is also a good source of such important minerals as iron, potassium and magnesium.

In addition to its role in protecting cells from damage and protecting the body from common pathogens, basil is believed to have important health effects on the heart and cardiovascular system. In addition, the high levels of vitamin A contained in basil make it important to maintaining good eyesight and healthy skin and hair.

Additional information: Basil is one of the easiest herbs to grow at home, and many people prefer the benefits of having a steady supply of fresh basil. There are many recipes that make full use of this aromatic herb, and fresh basil tends to provide a better taste the dried variety.

Of course the dried basil available in local grocery stores, health food stores and supermarkets also provides the many health benefits associated with this common herb. Dried basil is an excellent alternative to fresh for those who do not wish to grow their own. When choosing dried basil, however, it is important to choose those varieties that have undergone the least possible amount of processing. How herbs such as basil are processed can have a significant impact on both their nutritional value and their good taste.

Fresh basil should be chosen over the dried variety as much as possible, however, since the fresh variety is of superior flavor and nutrition. When choosing fresh basil from the supermarket, it is important to choose basil that is deep green and vibrant looking. In addition, the basil should not contain any yellow or dark spots.

Fresh basil can be stored in the refrigerator, either in its original packaging or in a dampened paper towel. Basil can also be frozen, either whole or chopped, as long as it is stored in an airtight container.

When purchasing dried basil, it is a good idea to seek out organically grown varieties, and to be sure that the herb has not been irradiated. Irradiated basil has been shown to lose some of its nutritional value, especially the healthy carotenoids that make it such a superfood.

Thyme

Classification: culinary herbs, edible

Origin: The herb known as thyme is native to Asia, southern Europe and the Mediterranean region. In addition to these traditional growing places, thyme is also widely cultivated throughout North America.

Thyme has been valued for thousands of years for its aromatic, culinary and medicinal uses. Thyme was even used by those in ancient Egypt as an embalming agent for deceased pharaohs.

The ancient Greeks valued thyme mainly for its aromatic properties, and thyme was frequently burned as incense in the temples of Greece. In addition, thyme was seen by the Greeks as a symbol of admiration and courage. This association of thyme with courage continued throughout the Middle Ages, and it was traditional for women to present their knights with a spring of thyme. Since at least the 16th century, thyme oil has been used as an antiseptic, both as a mouthwash and as a topical preparation.

Major benefits of thyme: Thyme has long been used in traditional medicine to treat chest problems and respiratory issues, including coughing, bronchitis, and chest congestion.   Recent research into these traditional uses of thyme has pinpointed the compounds that are responsible for these effects.   In particular, the volatile oil of thyme is known to include such healing compounds as borneol, carvacolo, geraniol and thymol.

Thymol is thought to be the most important and most medicinally valuable of the elements in thyme. The healthy effects of thymol have been well documented, and thymol has been shown to provide protection on a cellular level. In particular, DHA, an omega-3 fatty acid was increased as a result of supplementation with thyme in a recent study, and it is thought that this increased production of DHA is largely responsible for the cell protecting effects of this herb.

It is thought that the cell protecting benefits of thyme may be able to mitigate the effects of aging, and in addition thyme is known to be a food that is rich in antioxidants, and in the important mineral known as manganese.

In addition, thyme has been shown to have strong antimicrobial benefits, and the volatile oil components of thyme have been shown to be effective against a variety of harmful bacterial and fungal infections. Some of the microbes that these essential oils have been shown to fight include Staphalococcus aureus, Bacillus subtilis, Escherichia coli and Shigella sonnei.

Additional information: For many thousands of years, spices, herbs and other foodstuffs have been used to preserve foods, to provide much needed nutrients and to prevent contamination by harmful microbes.

Thyme has been shown to be one of the most nutrient dense of all spices, and it sports a truly impressive array of minerals, vitamins and other important nutrients. In addition, thyme provides a great flavor and is highly useful in a seemingly endless variety of recipes.

Whenever and wherever possible, it is best to choose fresh thyme over the dried herb. Fresh thyme will have a superior flavor, and it may have a superior nutrient content as well. The leaves of fresh thyme should appear fresh, and the leaves should be of a vibrant green-gray color. Thyme leaves should contain no yellowing or dark spots.

Fresh thyme can be stored refrigerated, either in a dampened paper towel or in its original packaging. When using dried thyme it is important to store it in a dark, dry and cool location, and the dried herb will keep in this way for up to six months.

Oregano

Classification: culinary herbs, edible

Origin: The herb known as oregano is native to northern Europe, but it grows throughout many regions of the world. Oregano has long been prized for its aroma and its strong taste, and the ancient Greeks and Romans used the herb as a symbol of happiness and joy. Oregano was held in such high esteem that brides in Greek and Roman society were often crowned with laurels of oregano.

Oregano has been cultivated in France ever since the Middle Ages, and it has been an important part of Mediterranean cooking for nearly as long. Oregano was almost unknown in the United States until early in the 20th century, when soldiers returning from Italy brought this fragrant herb back with them to the U.S.

Major benefits of oregano: Oregano is an herb known to have many important benefits, but one of the most significant of these health benefits may lie in the antibacterial properties of the herb. The volatile oils contained in oregano include thymol and carvacrol. Both of these volatile oils have been shown to help reduce the growth of bacteria, including such common bacteria as pseudomonas aeruginosa and staphylococcus aureus.

In Mexico, researchers have found the effects of oregano to be comparable to those of tinidazol, a prescription drug commonly used to treat infections from the amoeba known as giardia lamblia. This research actually found oregano to be superior to tinidazol in fighting this common infection.

In addition to its power as an antimicrobial agent, oregano is a potent source of antioxidant vitamins. The antioxidant vitamins contained in oregano are thought to play an important role in fighting cancer, heart disease and other common ailments. There is a great deal of study underway into the anticancer potential of oregano, and this ability to fight cancer may prove to be one of the most valuable benefits of this popular herb.

Oregano is one of the most antioxidant dense foods available, and this superfood has been shown to have more 42 times more antioxidant activity than apples, 30 times more antioxidants than potatoes and 12 times greater antioxidant value than oranges.

Additional information: It is generally better to choose fresh oregano instead of the dried varieties, since fresh oregano provides a more robust flavor. Leaves of fresh oregano should be a bright green color, and the stems of the plant should be firm to the touch. It is also important that the plant not contain any yellow or dark spots.

Fresh oregano is available in many supermarkets, but the freshest and most fragrant fresh oregano is often found at spice stores and natural grocers. For an even fresher source of oregano, why not grow it as part of an herb garden? Oregano is quite easy to grow indoors, and an herb garden can provide a ready source of fresh herbs at very low prices.

Fresh oregano is best kept refrigerated, and it is often helpful to wrap the fresh herb in a slightly damp paper towel. In addition, this fresh oregano can be frozen in airtight freezer containers. Fresh oregano can also be frozen using ice cube trays. These ice cube trays can be covered either with plain water or with fresh stock. These frozen oregano cubes can then be used to prepare soups and stews. Once dried, oregano can be kept in a tightly sealed container and stored in a dry, dark and cool location. Kept this way, dried oregano will last for up to six months.

Cinnamon

Classification: culinary herbs, edible

Origin: The spice known as cinnamon is one of the oldest in the entire world. In fact, cinnamon is mentioned several times in the Bible and it was used throughout ancient Egypt for a number of purposes. In addition to its use as a flavoring for various beverages and as a medicine, cinnamon was used as an embalming agents by the priests as they prepared the pharaohs for burial in the pyramids.

In these ancient cultures, cinnamon was valued more highly than gold, and around the same time cinnamon was receiving plenty of attention in China as well. The use of cinnamon in both Chinese cuisine and Chinese medicine is thought to date back at least to the year 2700 B.C.

The popularity of cinnamon continued to grow as the years passed, and it became one of the most important spices in the world of Medieval Europe. Cinnamon was one of the first commodities to be traded between the worlds of Europe and the Near East.

Today most commercial cinnamon is produced in Sri Lanka, India, Brazil, Madagascar, the countries of the Caribbean, China, Indonesia and Vietnam.

Major benefits of cinnamon: In many cultures around the world, the spice known as cinnamon has been used not just for its good taste but for its medicinal values as well. As a matter of fact, cinnamon has been highly valued as a traditional medicine for hundreds, if not thousands, of years.

One of the most important benefits of cinnamon is its promise in treating type-2 diabetes. A recent clinical study published in the journal Diabetes Care found that those diabetics who consumed half a teaspoon of cinnamon each day were able to significantly reduce their level of blood sugar.

The same study also found that those type 2 diabetes sufferers who consumed a half teaspoon of cinnamon a day also had lower levels of triglycerides, LDL (bad) cholesterol and total blood cholesterol.

In addition to its potential value at treating type 2 diabetes, cinnamon has long been used to improve digestion and to reduce the occurrence of stomach cramps, diarrhea, irritable bowel syndrome and other common digestive disorders. Many have found that adding cinnamon to the daily diet can improve digestion and reduce intestinal distress.

Cinnamon has also been shown to help reduce the pain of arthritis, and recent studies have suggested that cinnamon may contain important anti-inflammatory compounds. There is considerable anecdotal evidence that cinnamon is effective at reducing the pain associated with arthritis and other inflammatory diseases.

Additional information: Cinnamon has also been shown to help reduce joint pain and muscle stiffness, and those who consume cinnamon on a regular basis often report an improvement in their condition and relief from their pain.

Cinnamon may even be able to provide relief from menstrual cramping and similar discomfort. In traditional cultures, cinnamon has long been used to treat menstrual cramping and pain.

In addition, cinnamon acts as a blood thinner, and it may be able to provide better circulation. In this, cinnamon is thought to provide similar benefits to garlic, although its blood thinning properties are not as strong as those contained in garlic.

Cinnamon is thought to play a role in killing harmful bacteria as well, especially those associated with tooth decay and gum disease. In addition, cinnamon has shown effectiveness at killing such harmful microorganisms as E. coli.

Cinnamon is available in a variety of forms, including stick and powder. Cinnamon sticks have a longer shelf life, while the powdered form of cinnamon generally has a more robust flavor. If you can, it is important to smell the cinnamon, as quality cinnamon will have a sweet smell.

Both the Ceylon and Chinese varieties of cinnamon may be labeled as cinnamon, so it is important to know the difference between the two varieties. Ceylon cinnamon provides a sweeter and more refined taste than the Chinese variety. The Ceylon variety of cinnamon is generally harder to come by, however, and it may be necessary to visit a spice store or ethnic supermarket to obtain quality Ceylon cinnamon.

When purchasing cinnamon, no matter what the variety, it is important to be sure that the spice has not been irradiated, as radiation has been shown to reduce the concentration of vitamin C and carotenoids in cinnamon.

Cinnamon is best stored in a glass container with a tight seal, and it should be kept in a dark, dry and cool location for longer shelf life. Ground cinnamon which is properly stored can last for up to six months, while fresh cinnamon sticks can last up to one year when properly stored. The shelf life of both cinnamon sticks and powdered cinnamon can be extended by keeping it in the refrigerator.

Mint

Classification: culinary herbs, edible

Origin: Mint has long been grown in many places around the world, from Europe to the Middle East to India, and this herb has been enjoyed for its medicinal, aromatic and culinary properties alike.

Mint is an herb with a very long history indeed, and it is even celebrated in a famous Greek myth in which a nymph named Minthe was turned into a plant by Persephone, who was jealous of Minthe's relationship with her husband Pluto. While Pluto was unable to reverse the spell cast by his wife, he did provide Minthe with a sweet smell, and it is this sweet aroma that makes mint so attractive today.

This wonderful aroma has long made mint a favorite herb for use in the home, and societies from the Middle East to Europe and India have long stewed mint to clear the air in their homes and in their temples. In addition, mint has traditionally been used as a symbol of welcome and hospitality. In ancient Greece, it was customary to rub mint leaves on the dining table as a welcome to guests, and Middle Eastern societies have long welcomed their guests with fresh mint tea.

Major benefits of mint: Mint is an herb with a long history in the world of traditional medicine, and mint has long been used to soothe digestion and to reduce stomach aches and similar problems.

Mint leaves and mint teas have been shown to reduce the symptoms of irritable bowel syndrome and other digestive problems. The instance of irritable bowel syndrome and similar conditions are on the rise, and mint remains one of the most effective ways to treat this common condition.

In addition, mint has been shown to be quite effective at reducing the growth of many types of harmful bacteria and fungi. These antibacterial and antifungal properties of mint are the subject of much ongoing research. In addition, mint is thought to have the ability to reduce the symptoms of asthma and allergies as well.

Mint may even provide important anticancer benefits. Like many other superfoods, mint is thought to provide important protection against many common forms of cancer. Mint is known to contain an important phytonutrient known as perillyl alcohol, a compound that has been shown in animal studies to protect against the formation of colon, skin and lung cancer. While additional research still needs to be done, the results so far look quite promising.

Mint has also been shown to provide beneficial effects for those suffering from asthma. This effect is thought to be due to the presence of rosmarinic acid found in mint. In addition to the ability to neutralize free radicals, this valuable compound has been found to block the production of certain inflammatory chemicals such as leukotrienes. This blocking of leukotrienes is thought to provide protection against asthma attacks. In addition, mint has been shown to have a positive impact on allergies and similar conditions.

Additional information: Mint can be used in many ways, but one of the most popular ways to use it is in a tea. To make a good mint tea, one or two teaspoons of dried mint leaves are used, and hot, but not boiling water is poured over those leaves. The mixture must then be covered to prevent the valuable volatile oils from evaporating. The mixture is allowed to steep for ten minutes, and then drained as used as a delicious and therapeutic tea. This mint tea is often used to treat stomach aches and other common stomach problems. When drinking mint tea for stomach ailments, the recommended dosage is three to four cups of tea per day.

In addition to being used as a tea, mint can also be used in capsule form. There are many enteric-coated capsules that are made with fresh mint leaves, and these enteric capsules can be a good choice for those who suffer from nausea and similar conditions. Both the tea and the capsules work well, and the choice is entirely up to you.

Licorice

Classification: culinary herb, edible

Origin: Licorice, known to science as glycyrrhizin glabra, is a member of the pea family that is widely cultivated throughout Greece and Turkey. The key therapeutic compound contained in licorice is glycyrrhizin, and this compound is found in the underground stem of the tall purple flowered shrub.

In addition to the glycyrrhizin, licorice is thought to contain hundreds of other healthful ingredients, including flavonoids and plant estrogens known as phytoestrogens. Licorice is thought to have a number of healing properties, including anti-inflammatory properties and the ability to sooth stomach upset.

Major benefits of licorice: Licorice has long been used to treat stomach upset, and this remains one of the chief benefits of licorice. In addition, licorice is currently being studied for everything from its ability to reduce coughs to its possible use as an anticancer agent.

The glycyrrhizin contained in licorice is known to have many important benefits to the human body, and it is known to be useful in treating a wide variety of ailments. For instance, licorice appears to have the ability to boost the immune system by increasing levels of interferon, an important compound in fighting viral attacks. In addition, licorice root contains many powerful antioxidant vitamins, as well as many important and healthful phytoestrogens. These plant-based estrogens are known to provide some of the same functions as the natural estrogens found in the body.

In addition, licorice helps to protect the digestive system from corrosive stomach acids through the stimulation of substances that coat the esophagus and the stomach. This characteristic of licorice makes it useful for a number of different ailments, including many digestive and intestinal disorders.

Licorice may also be valuable at treating and controlling various respiratory conditions, including chest congestion, coughing and sore throats. Licorice is thought to help loosen and thin the mucus in the airways, resulting in a more productive cough and thus a reduction in phlegm and mucus. Licorice is also known to help reduce bronchial spasms and to soothe sore throats. Licorice is even thought to help fight the viruses that cause recurrent respiratory conditions.

Another important potential benefit of licorice is the ability to reduce the symptoms of chronic fatigue syndrome and fibromyalgia. It is thought that this effect is produced by enhancing cortisol activity. Conditions like fibromyalgia and chronic fatigue syndrome are known to be sensitive to cortisol levels, thus the effect of licorice on cortisol is thought to provide relief from these troubling conditions.

Licorice is also thought to protect the liver and promote healing in the organ as well. It is even thought that the anti-inflammatory properties of licorice may be able to soothe the liver inflammation associated with hepatitis. In addition, licorice also helps to fight the virus responsible for hepatitis, and the antioxidants it contains help to promote overall liver health.

Additional information: Licorice is often combined with other herbs and added to herbal blends, and licorice is particularly effective at disguising the bitterness of many herbal remedies.

Licorice is available in a variety of different forms, including wafers, tinctures, tablets, liquids, dried herbs, teas, creams, lozenges and capsules. For licorice products that contain glycyrrhizin, it is important to look for preparations that have been standardized to contain a 22% concentration of glycyrrhizinic acid or glycrrhizin.

Most disorders that respond to licorice respond well to 200 mg of standardized extract three times daily, or 20 to 45 drops of liquid medication three times per day. For coughs and chest congestion, the traditional remedy is to drink one cup of licorice tea three times each day. This licorice tea is made by pouring eight ounces of very hot but not boiling water over two teaspoons of dried herb. This mixture is then allowed to steep for 10 minutes and then strained.

A blended herbal tea used for coughs can be made by steeping one teaspoon each of dried licorice and slippery elm in very hot water. This tea is drunk three times per day, but it should be continued for no longer than three weeks.

Bilberry

Classification: supplements, edible

Origin: The bilberry is known to the world of science as actinium myrtillus, and it is a member of the blueberry family. Like the blueberry, the bilberry is blue in color and sweet in taste.

The bilberry bush is a shrubby perennial that grows wild in the meadows and forests of many places in Europe and Western Asia, as well as the Rocky Mountain regions of the United States and Canada. The bilberry is related to the cranberry, huckleberry and blueberry, and the fruit is of a similar appearance.

Major benefits of bilberry: For many years, the bilberry has been used in traditional medicine, and the leaves of the bilberry bush are known to have important healing properties as well.

One of the most significant benefits of the bilberry is the ability to enhance vision, particularly night vision. As far back as World War II, those fighter pilots who consumed large quantities of bilberries claimed to have better night vision, and many modern studies have backed this up. In addition, the bilberry has been shown to have the ability to slow many degenerative diseases of the eye, and the compounds contained in the bilberry may have the ability to improve visual acuity as well.

Other traditional uses of the bilberry included its use to treat diarrhea. As far back as the sixteenth century, the bilberry was combined with honey in order to make a syrup solution known as rob. This rob syrup was traditionally used to treat diarrhea and other digestive problems.

Bilberry is also thought to strengthen collagen, a protein responsible for the health of connective tissue, and it is thought to provide important benefits to the health of blood vessels as well. The compounds contained in the bilberry, specifically compounds known as anthocyanosides, have been shown to help fortify the walls of blood vessels, thereby increasing the flow of blood and improving circulation.

Bilberry is also known to be quite effective at soothing sore throats, and drinking or gargling with a cooled tea made with dried bilberries has proven to be very soothing to those suffering from sore or inflamed mouths and throats.

It is the eye, however, that is thought to benefit the most from the consumption of bilberry and bilberry containing supplements. For many years bilberry has been used to treat night blindness, and to reduce the affect of glare on daytime vision. In addition, it is thought that bilberry may play a role in preventing macular degeneration and other eye diseases associated with aging.

The compounds in bilberry may also help to slow down the formation of cataracts, another eye problem often associated with aging. It is thought that the high concentration of vitamin E and vitamin A in bilberries may account for this eye protective benefit.

In addition to its ability to improve vision and prevent its degeneration, those who eat bilberry on a regular basis have often noted a reduction in varicose veins. The active compounds contained in bilberry are thought to improve circulation and increase blood flow, therefore reducing the appearance of varicose veins and lessening their severity.

Additional information: The bilberry is known to contain large amounts of phytochemicals, and these phytochemicals are thought to have the ability to help lower blood pressure, reduce the formation of blood clots and to provide a greater blood supply to the nervous system. In addition, some scientific studies have suggested that the antioxidants contained in the fruit of the bilberry bush may be up to fifty times as effective as vitamin E and up to ten times as valuable as vitamin C. In addition, bilberry may be effective at reducing vascular insufficiency, and it is thought to work in the same way as horse chestnut and ginko biloba.

The bilberry is available in many varieties, including fresh bilberries and extracts in capsule and pill forms. It is important to buy bilberry, whether in fresh or pill form, from only the highest quality sources.

As with other foods and supplements, how the bilberry is harvested and processed can have a significant impact on both its nutritional value and its taste. It is important that the bilberry be harvested at the peak of ripeness, and that it is processed using the most modern state of the art manufacturing methods.

Milk Thistle

Classification: supplements

Origin: The plant known as milk thistle grows throughout the world, including in many parts of the North American continent. Milk thistle grows wild in many parts of the world, and it is also cultivated for its medicinal value. The scientific community knows milk thistle as silybum marianum, and its active compounds are referred to as siilymarin. Concentrated stores of silymarin are located in the black fruit of the plant, which are harvested at the end of the summer. In fact, the milk thistle plant is a member of the sunflower family, although its flowers are not yellow like those of the traditional sunflower.

Major benefits of milk thistle: What makes milk thistle a superfood is its ability to treat a variety of liver problems, and milk thistle has been used for this purpose for more than two thousand years. Traditional healers have long been acquainted with the liver healing properties of the milk thistle plant, and modern science has discovered that milk thistle has the ability to stimulate the flow of bile from the liver. It is this bile stimulation that is thought to account for the ability of milk thistle to treat a number of liver ailments. Milk thistle also seems to be effective at protecting the liver from damage. In Europe milk thistle is used to treat a variety of liver ailments, form hepatitis to cirrhosis.

Milk thistle is also thought to help reduce the damage to the liver caused by excessive alcohol consumption. Excessive consumption of alcohol is known to reduce the concentration of glutathione, a substance that can reduce toxins in the liver. The depletion of this important element can cause living scarring, a condition known as cirrhosis. Not only is milk thistle known to boost the production of glutathione, but it is also able to repair previous damage to the liver by promoting the growth of new liver cells.

The bile secreting effects of milk thistle may also be responsible for the ability of the plant to aid in digestion. In addition, milk thistle has shown promise in treating other ailments as well, including gallstones, allergies, high cholesterol and even skin cancer.

Milk thistle is thought to have strong antioxidant properties, and it is these antioxidant properties that may be responsible for the protective benefits of this plant.

In the world of modern medicine, there is an injectible form of milk thistle that is used as a powerful antidote to the effects of poison mushrooms. In addition, extract of milk thistle has been studied as a possible treatment for the liver damage that often accompanies chemotherapy treatment. It is thought that milk thistle extract may have the ability to speed up the elimination of toxins from the body, and this may help to mitigate chemotherapy induced liver damage.

In addition, milk thistle is thought to have strong anti-inflammatory benefits, and this may make it useful in controlling the skin rash associated with psoriasis and at slowing down the growth of abnormal skin cells.

Additional information: Milk thistle is found in a variety of different preparations, such as tablets, capsules, soft gels and tinctures. Those who wish to use milk thistle to treat liver problems should find a standardized extract of between 400 to 600 mg, and spread the daily dose in three equal portions.

Milk thistle tea is often seen as well, but in general the concentrations of silymaria contained in milk thistle tea are of no medicinal value. While the tea can be enjoyable, it is important to use other preparations for medicinal benefit.

Echinacea

Classification: supplements

Origin: The herb we know as Echinacea, also called the purple coneflower, actually consists of nine distinct species, but only three varieties are used in herbal medicine. Those three varieties are:

- ➢ Echinacea engustifolia
- ➢ Echinacea pallida
- ➢ Echinacea purpurea

The herb known as Echinacea is native to the plains of the North American continent, and it has been cultivated for many years and used in traditional medicine and natural healing.

Major benefits of Echinacea: The herb known as Echinacea is best known as a possible cold fighter and immune system booster. While the results of various clinical studies have so far been inconclusive, many of those who use Echinacea on a regular basis report a lower incidence of colds, flu and other infections than before they began taking the supplement. One effect of

Echinacea seems to be its ability to boost the production of interferon, an important substance used by the body to fight viral infections.

When taking Echinacea to fight an existing cold, flu or other condition, it is important to take the herb at the first sign of cold or flu. Echinacea is thought to have the ability to shorten the duration of these common illnesses, but it is important to take the supplement when the first symptoms appear.

In addition to its role as a possible cold and flu fighter, Echinacea is being studied as a way to fight common respiratory ailments like bronchitis, sinusitis and strep throat. These common illnesses often recur year after year and Echinacea is thought to have the power to prevent their recurrence. As with colds and flu, it is best to take the herb at the first sign of illness.

Echinacea is also being studied as a possible way to speed up the healing of cuts and wounds to the skin, as well as a way to reduce inflammation. Conditions that have been successfully treated with Echinacea supplements include burns, cuts, scrapes and sores, as well as abscesses, boils, canker sores and eczema. Echinacea can be applied directly to the skin in the form of a cream or taken orally to promote a healthy immune system response to skin issues.

Echinacea has even shown promise at treating one of the most baffling conditions of modern life – Chronic Fatigue Syndrome. While science is still unsure of the origins and causes of CFS, many of those who suffer from this puzzling condition have reported relief from their symptoms when taking Echinacea supplements.

Additional information: Various parts of the plant produce Echinacea, including the flowers, leaves, stems and roots. These are all used in the many different commercial preparations on the market. It is important to be sure that the Echinacea preparation you buy contain pure ingredients in sufficient quantities to be effective against colds, flu, infections and other conditions. It is important, therefore, to carefully read the label when choosing Echinacea supplements, and to buy your supplements only from quality and reputable companies.

Echinacea supplements are available in quite a number of forms, including soft gels, capsules, tablets, ointments, liquids and tinctures. In addition, the Echinacea herb can be purchased in a dried form and brewed into a soothing and healing tea. There are also a number of creams containing Echinacea that can be rubbed directly into the skin to promote healing and improve the condition of the skin.

Ginseng

Classification: supplements

Origin: Ginseng is native to the Siberian plain and to many parts of Asia. Ginseng has long been used as an energy tonic in traditional Chinese medicine, and its use dates back thousands of years.

Major benefits of ginseng: While the many health benefits of ginseng have long been known to the world of traditional Chinese medicine, the Western world has been slower to accept the healing power of this important herb.

One of the most significant benefits of ginseng is its ability to reduce stress in men and women alike. In many clinical trials, those taking regular supplements of ginseng reported being able to tolerate higher levels of physical and emotional stress.

In addition, ginseng is thought to be highly effective in fighting fatigue, in fighting off colds and the flu and in enhancing the performance of memory.

Ginseng is known to contain a great many compounds that are unique to this herb, and many of these compounds are thought to have a profound effect on the adrenal glands. The adrenal glands are small glands that rest on top of the kidneys, and their job is to secrete hormones that are useful in fighting physical and emotional stress. It is thought that ginseng has the ability to enhance the ability to fight both physical and emotional stress through their effect on the adrenal glands.

For this reason, ginseng is thought to be able to prevent the many diseases that have stress as their cause. These stress related conditions include heart disease and stroke, and even some forms of cancer.

Ginseng is also thought to play a role in the treatment of chronic fatigue syndrome. This condition has been one of the most puzzling to science, and there is no pharmaceutical cure for this syndrome. Ginseng is one of the few herbs that has shown promise at relieving the symptoms of chronic fatigue syndrome.

Additional information: In addition, many who have taken ginseng on a regular basis report being able to better withstand physical labor, suggesting that ginseng has a strong effect on the body as well as the mind. Many who use ginseng report the ability to work at higher speed and with greater levels of accuracy. In addition, ginseng may help people adapt to heat, high altitudes and low oxygen conditions more easily. Ginseng is also thought to help enhance concentration and mental alertness.

Traditional Chinese medicine held that ginseng was a strong aphrodisiac, and many feel that ginseng has the ability to enhance fertility in both men and women. In addition to enhancing fertility, ginseng may have the ability to treat symptoms of menopause.

Ginseng is available over the counter in a number of different preparations, and in a number of different stores, including grocery stores, supermarkets, health food stores and Internet retailers. When buying ginseng, it is important to choose those made with the purest ingredients, and to choose those manufactured to the highest quality standards using state of the art equipment.

While allergies to and side effects of ginseng are quite rare, it is important to always be on the lookout for any adverse effects of ginseng supplementation. Ginseng supplements are quite safe at the recommended doses, and these supplements can generally be used for even long periods of time without adverse health effects.

On rare occasions, however, mild diarrhea has been known to occur. If this symptom does not clear up within a week or two, it could indicate either that you are sensitive to ginseng or that the dosage should be reduced.

At extremely high doses of ginseng, those exceeding 900 mg per day, insomnia, irritability, nervousness and anxiety have been known to occur. As with all supplements, it is important to discuss the supplements you are taking with your physician. It is important for your doctor to have a clear picture of all medications, including prescription drugs, over the counter medications and herbal remedies that you are taking.

St John's Wort

Classification: supplements

Origin: The herb that has come to be known as St John's Wort is known to science as hypericum perforatum, and it was of course named in honor of St. John the Baptist. The golden flowers of St. John's Wort traditionally bloom in June, which was the month of St. John the Baptist's birth. The term "wort" means, "plant", therefore St John's Wort is actually St Johns plant.

The herb known as St John's Wort is a perennial, meaning that it will spring back to life year after year on only a single planting. St. John's Wort grows wild, particularly in Europe, and it has been used for its medicinal benefits for perhaps thousands of years.

St John's Wort has been used for thousands of years, with its use in traditional medicine dating back at least 2400 years. As a matter of fact, the founder of the science of medicine, Hippocrates, is known to have used St. John's Wort to cure such diverse diseases as hemorrhages, dysentery, jaundice, tuberculosis, colds, flu and insomnia.

Major benefits of St. John's Wort: The herb known as St. John's Wort is perhaps best known, however, for treating issues like depression and anxiety. Depression and anxiety continue to be serious health concerns throughout the country, and unfortunately many of those who suffer from such conditions resist seeking the professional help they need.

Fortunately for those people, there are a number of natural and herbal remedies for depression, anxiety and related conditions, and St. John's Wort has shown real promise in treating these serious medical problems. Many clinical studies have backed up the ability of St John's Wort to improve mood and many people have found real relief from using this herbal remedy.

St John's Wort has shown so much promise in treating anxiety and depression that it is routinely prescribed for these conditions in many European countries, and it continues to be used in traditional Chinese medicine as it has for thousands of years.

Studies of St John's Wort have found that this herb contains a unique combination of ingredients, including hypericin. Hypericin seems to be the most important of the many compounds contained in St John's wort, and it is thought to react with certain brain chemicals, therefore providing a calming effect and a level of emotional comfort in many people. In fact, it is thought that St John's Wort has much the same effect on these brain chemicals as many common prescription medications used to treat depression and anxiety.

In addition to its effect on depression and anxiety, St John's Wort is thought to provide relief from insomnia, and possibly even to improve cardiac circulation and the health of the cardiovascular system.

Additional information: In the United States, there are a great many different preparations of St John's Wort, made by a number of different companies and available in a number of different strengths.

When used orally, St. John's Wort is most often taken in capsule or tablet form. The most effective preparation of St. John's Wort seems to be a standardized dose of 300 mg containing a 0.3 concentration of hypericin. The suggested dosage ranges from 2 to 12 capsules or tablets per day, depending on the condition being treated and its severity.

In addition to tablets and capsules, St. John's Wort is also available as a tea. This St. John's Wort tea is made by mixing two teaspoons of the dried herb with hot water, then allowing it to steep for 10 minutes. After the tea has steeped, it is strained, and then mixed with honey or sugar for a tasty and effective drink.

St. John's Wort can also be infused with olive oil and used as massage oil. This preparation is particularly useful at relieving inflammation and joint pain. In addition, this massage oil may be good at speeding the healing of wounds and bruises to the skin.

As with all supplements, it is important to notify your family physician of all medications and herbal supplements you are taking. It is important for your doctor to have a clear picture of all medications you are taking to treat anxiety, depression and other conditions. This means not only informing your doctor about the prescription medications you are taking, but keeping him or her apprised of all over the counter preparations and herbal supplements as well.

Astragalus

Classification: supplements

Origin: Astragalus is native to the continent of Asia, and it has been one of the most popular energy tonics in Oriental medicine for many years.

Astragalus, known to science as astragaluls membranaceus, is actually a member of the legume family, and it has been safely used in traditional medicine for thousands of years. This plant is native to the central and western regions of Asia, particularly Korea, China and Taiwan, and this superfood seems to have the rare ability to boost certain functions of the immune system while suppressing others. Few other foods have this ability, and that is what makes astagalus so special and so exciting.

Astragalus (Astragalus membranaceus) is a member of the legume family and is considered an adaptogenic herb in traditional Chinese medicine, where it has been safely used for centuries. Native to central and western Asia, specifically China, Korea and Taiwan, Astragalus offers a unique benefit found in very few herbs - it seems to selectively support immune system function by stimulating certain immune functions and

The superfood known as astragalus has been used for thousands of years for its important health benefits, and it is an important element of traditional medicine and alternative medicine.

While modern science has been slower to catch on to the many benefits of this superfood, many studies are now underway into the many health benefits of astragalus, and they have suggested that this supplement has an important role to play in improving the function of the immune system.

Major benefits of Astragalus: One of the most important medicinal effects of astragals seems to be its ability to boost the immune system, and a recent study found that astragals aids in improving the function of the immune system by increasing T-cell counts.

The most important active ingredient of astragals is a compound known as astragalan

B. Astragalan B is a compound known as a polysaccharide, it is known to help bind cholesterol and to help the body fight off microbes and other invaders. In addition, astragals and the astragalan B it contains is also thought to help speed the cleansing of toxins from the body.

While studies are still ongoing, it is thought that astragals may turn out to be potentially very valuable to those patients living with cancer and AIDS. In traditional Chinese medicine, astragalus has long been used in cancer patients to improve immune response following chemotherapy and radiation treatments. As a result, the Chinese often prescribe astragals as a compliment to chemotherapy and radiation treatments. In addition, astragalus is often used as an adjunct to traditional therapies for both cancer and AIDS.

Astragalus is also thought to help the lungs and the spleen function more efficiently, and it is also used to treat a variety of vascular diseases and to support circulation, lower blood pressure levels and keep blood sugar levels in check.

In addition, astragalus has also been shown to improve a healthy cardiovascular system by protecting the membranes of cells from the damage done by free radicals. The antioxidant properties of astragalus are thought to provide important protective benefits to the heart.

Additional information: In addition to these important benefits, astragals may even prove to be a natural replacement for Viagra and other similar drugs. When combined with other traditional medicines like yohimbe and cordyceps, astragalus is thought to activate sexual function and help keep everything functioning smoothly. So not only is astragal a powerful energy tonic but it may be an excellent aphrodisiac as well.

The most unique feature of astragalus is probably its ability to selectively support the function of the immune system by stimulating some immune system functions while depressing other functions of the immune system. One reason for this selective immune system power may be the high selenium content astragalus contains. Selenium is a vital trace mineral, and unfortunately many of the world soils have become deficient in selenium. This makes the consumption of foods rich in selenium, such as astragalus, even more important.

Astragalus also contains vital compounds like polysaccharides and flavonoids, which are known to support the health of the immune system while minimizing the harmful effects of free radicals on cell membranes. This important superfood has shown the ability to stimulate the so-called resting immune system, increasing the activity of resting immune system cells. In addition, new research has revealed that astragalus is able to support the production of macrophages, immunoglobulin, natural killer cells and T cells, which form the core of the army known as the immune system.

Ginko

Classification: supplements

Origin: Ginko has been cultivated in China and other Asian countries for thousands of years, and it has been used in traditional Chinese medicine for almost as long. For nearly 2800 years, ginko has been used to treat a wide variety of ailments. Ginko is derived from the tree of the same name, and the tree is native to many parts of Asia.

The plant was first brought to the Europe in the 17th century, and it is now used throughout the world. Ginko biloba is one of the most heavily researched herbs in the entire world, and it is the subject of a great deal of ongoing research.

The ginko biloba tree has been around for a long time indeed, with estimates that it has been growing on the earth for between 150 and 200 million years. For thousands of years, ginko has been used to improve blood flow, increase sexual energy, improve longevity and increase overall well being.

Major benefits of Ginko: Ginko has a number of important health benefits, including the ability to maintain normal blood circulation, proper function of blood vessels, reducing tissue damage and maintaining proper levels of glucose and oxygen in the blood.

In addition, ginko contains a number of very valuable antioxidant vitamins, including the all-important flavonoids. These nutrients are a valuable way to combat the damage done by free radicals.

It is the effects on the blood that provide ginko with its most important benefits, however. Ginko is thought to have the ability to increase blood flow to the brain, and this may in turn be able to boost memory functions and aid in overall brain health.

Ginko also acts as a blood thinner, and it is thought to interfere with what is known as platelet activating factor (PAF). It is this PAF, which is thought to be part of the cause of asthma, hearing problems, heart disease and of skin conditions such as psoriasis.

In addition to its physical benefits, ginko is thought to have significant benefits on emotional health as well, and many people have found that ginko has the ability to reduce anxiety and tension. For many people, ginko seems to act to boost mood and restore energy.

Additional information: Ginko preparations are found in a large number of forms, including pills, tablets, capsules and soft gels. Since ginko is one of the most widely manufactured herbal supplements on the market, it is important to buy only the highest quality preparations, made by the most reputable and established manufacturers.

It is also important that the manufacturing process completely remove the toxic element of the ginko leaf, also known as ginkgolic acid. Processed ginko preparations should contain no more than 5 parts per million (ppm) of ginkgolic acid, and the vast majority of commercial ginko on the market is well under this limit.

Flax (flax seed oil)

Classification: supplements, edible

Origin: Flax seeds and flaxseed oil has been known throughout history. While flaxseed oil first originated in ancient Mesopotamia, but flax seeds have been known since the Stone Age. The ancient Greeks were among the first to use the flax seed in cooking, and both the ancient Greeks and the ancient Romans prized the flax seed and its flaxseed oil for its health benefits and its good taste. Following the collapse of the Roman civilization the cultivation of the flax plant declined substantially.

It was the emperor Charlemagne who would return flax seeds to their former high position in culinary culture. Charlemagne was impressed not only with the culinary and medicinal uses of the flax plant but with its usefulness as a fiber as well. Flaxseed fibers can be woven into linen and Charlemagne pass laws that required both the cultivation of the flax plant and the consumption of flax seeds and flaxseed oil. As a result of Charlemagne's efforts, flax seeds and flaxseed oil become widely used throughout Europe.

Flax plants were not cultivated in North America until the 17th century, when flax plants were planted in Canada. To this day, Canada remains the leading producer of flax seeds and flaxseed oil.

Major benefits of flax and flax seed oil: Flax seeds and flaxseed oil are rich in an omega-3 fatty acid known as alpha linolenic acid, which is a precursor to the beneficial fat known as EPA found in fish. This fatty acid provides many of the same benefits to those found in the best fish, including important benefits such as protecting the heart from damage. Omega-3 fatty acids are among the most important heart protectors, and flaxseed oil contains abundant quantities of these important fatty acids.

In addition, flaxseed oil is thought to provide important anti-inflammatory benefits, making it useful for such conditions as asthma, osteoarthritis, rheumatoid arthritis and even migraine headaches. Flaxseed oil may even be protective against many forms of cancer, and flaxseed oil is being studied for its possible cancer fighting properties.

The omega-3 fatty acids contained in flaxseed oil are also thought to play an important role in protecting cell membranes from damage. These cell membranes represent the cell's best protection, and they serve to allow in needed nutrients while keeping out harmful microbes and accumulated wastes.

Flax seeds also provide a rich source of dietary fiber, thought to play an important role in preventing cancer, heart disease and many other common diseases. Dietary fiber is thought to play an especially important role in preventing colon cancer, and those at highest risk for this disease are urged to eat plenty of fiber rich foods, including flax seeds and flaxseed oil.

Flax seeds and flaxseed oil are also thought to be effective at warding off the chronic and annoying condition known as dry eyes. Dry eye syndrome is thought to affect over 10 million Americans every year, and the traditional treatment of artificial tears is able to provide only temporary relief. Recent studies have shown that the consumption of flaxseed oil may be able to reduce the incidence and severity of dry eye syndrome.

Additional information: Flax seeds can be purchased either as whole seeds or in ground varieties. Although ground flax seeds are easier to use and more convenient, the whole seeds have a longer shelf life.

Whole flax seeds are available both in pre-packaged containers and in bulk bins in many natural grocery stores. When purchasing flax seeds from bins, it is important to make sure that the bins provide a secure cover, and that the flax seeds they contain are fresh. It is also important to store whole flax seeds in an airtight container, and to keep them in a dark, dry and cool place. Flax seeds stored in this manner can keep for several months.

Ground flax seeds are available in both refrigerated and non-refrigerated varieties. It is important to buy ground flax seeds in vacuum packed containers and to refrigerate them after the package has been opened. It is important to keep ground flax seeds refrigerated in order to prevent them from becoming rancid.

Like ground flax seeds, flaxseed oil is quite perishable and is best purchased in opaque bottles that have been kept refrigerated. Quality flaxseed oil will have a sweet and nutty flavor. Flaxseed oil should never be used for cooking, but only added to foods after they have been heated.

Spirulina

Classification: supplements

Origin: The superfood known as spirulina has been eaten for centuries and indigenous people have long known of the many health benefits imparted by this ancient algae. Modern medicine, however, has been much slower to embrace this valuable foodstuff, and scientific research into the health effects of spirulina began a mere three decades ago.

Spirulina is one of those foods that simply seems too good to be true. The algae commonly known as Spirulina, is well known for both its high protein content and its chlorophyll content. Both the chlorophyll and the protein of this superfood provide incredible health benefits for those who eat it.

In addition, spirulina is one of the richest sources of vitamins, minerals and amino acids, making it one of the most nutrient dense of all foods. There is no wonder why this well kept secret, known so well to ancient peoples, is becoming better known year by year.

Major benefits of spirulina: Modern research into the health benefits of spirulina has focused on five important benefits of this superfood. Specifically, spirulina appears to be able to:

> ➢ Strengthen the power of the immune system to fight disease
> ➢ Maintain healthy levels of cholesterol and improve the balance of good and bad cholesterol
> ➢ Support overall good cardiovascular function
> ➢ Improve the health of the gastrointestinal system
> ➢ Improve the natural detoxification and cleansing process of the body
> ➢ Provides strong antioxidant protection and anticancer benefits.

One of the things that makes Spirulina such a powerful superfood is its strong concentration of nutrients. Spirulina is high in protein, and it also contains high concentrations of vitamin B12, beta-carotene and iron. In addition, spirulina contains high concentrations of valuable compounds known as phytonutrients. It is these phytonutrients that are thought to play a vital role in preventing such killers as heart disease and cancer.

In addition, spirulina is rich in the natural antioxidants called carotenoids, which are vital to promoting cellular health. This cell health promotion is also thought to be responsible for many of the anticancer benefits of spirulina. In addition, spirulina contains chlorophyll, which is very good at detoxifying the body and cleansing it of the pollution in the environment.

Perhaps the most significant benefit of spirulina is its well-known ability to give a much-needed boost to the immune system. Much of the research into this important superfood has centered on its important role as an immune system stimulant. This ability to stimulate and enhance the immune system means that it may be able to help the body ward off dangerous pathogens naturally. This ability to naturally fight viruses, fungi and bacteria is becoming even more important as many common microbes develop immunity to even the strongest antibiotics.

Keeping the body healthy and the immune system strong are well known as the best way to avoid infection and retain good health. Those with a strong immune system will be able to fight off bacteria and viruses that those with a weakened immune system would easily fall victim to.

Have you ever wondered why several people can be exposed to the same pathogens and some get sick while others do not? You have probably seen this scenario play out at your workplace or your child's school. A roomful of people can be exposed to the same germs. Some get sick within a day or two, while others never miss a beat. The secret is a strong immune system. The stronger the immune system, the less likely you will be to succumb to illness. This is why the ability of spirulina to boost the immune system is so important.

It is thought that spirulina provides these immune system effects through the ability to bolster the natural killer cell functions of the body. Due to this mechanism it is thought that spirulina may be able to suppress both cancer and viral infections, and this is the subject of lots of research at the moment.

Some have even speculated that the higher spirulina consumption in Japan and Korea may be at least partially responsible for the lower incidence of HIV and AIDS in those countries. The speculation is that the immune boosting ability of this superfood may be able to fight this deadly infection.

Additional information: Spirulina is one of the most powerful of all the superfoods, but it is important that it be harvested, processed and packaged properly to retain its strong nutritional value. That is why it is so important to buy spirulina supplements only from the highest quality manufacturers, those who use state of the art harvesting, processing and packaging technology.

Boswellia

Classification: supplements

Origin: The fact that boswellia is also known as Indian frankincense provides an important clue to its origin, and in fact boswellia is native to the Indian subcontinent. Boswellia is derived from the boswellia serrata tree, which grows wild in the hills of the Indian subcontinent.

Indian healers have long used this "Indian frankincense" to treat a number of conditions, including inflammation and joint problems. In addition, boswellia is thought to be effective at treating back pain and some intestinal disorders as well. Boswellia is thought to provide many of the pain relieving and anti-inflammatory benefits of traditional prescription and over the counter pain relievers, without the stomach upset that can often accompany these medications.

The gummy resin of the tree is known as salai guggal, and many commercial preparations made from this purified extract and packaged in creams and pills are used to reduce inflammation and reduce the pain associated with both osteoarthritis and rheumatoid arthritis.

Major benefits of boswellia: For thousands of years Indian healers have used the gummy resin derived from the bark of the boswellia serrata tree for its strong anti-inflammatory benefits.

In the world of modern medicine, there are a great many preparations made with boswellia, and these preparations have shown real promise in reducing the inflammation associated with both rheumatoid arthritis and osteoarthritis. Boswellia preparations are available in both pills and creams, but the creams are most often used to reduce the inflammation associated with arthritis.

In addition to its effectiveness, boswellia has an important benefit over traditional non-steroidal anti-inflammatory (NSAID) drugs, and that is the fact that it does not cause stomach irritation like those drugs do.

In addition to its usefulness as an anti-arthritis preparation, boswellia has been found to be effective against chronic back pain and other inflammatory conditions. Both the oral and cream preparations of boswellia have proven effective at reducing lower back pain.

Additional information: Boswellia is available in many different preparations, including capsules, tablets and many topical creams. The topical varieties of boswellia are particularly effective against the pain of arthritis and at treating back pain. When using boswellia cream, a pea-sized amount of the cream should be rubbed into the affected area and treatment should be repeated every four to six hours as needed.

When choosing boswellia preparations, it is important to choose those products that have been standardized to a 60% concentration of boswellic acids. It is these boswellic acids that are thought to provide the therapeutic effects, so it is important to choose those preparations that contain a therapeutic level concentration of these healing compounds.

While side effects from boswellia are rare, on occasion diarrhea, nausea and skin rashes have been reported. Those who experience such side effects should discontinue their use of the supplement and notify their doctor. It is also important to consult with your family physician when using boswellia preparations to treat arthritis and other inflammatory diseases. It is important for your physician to have information about all medications you are taking, including over the counter medications and herbal remedies.

Conclusion

The superfoods listed in this document are among the most powerful and nutrient dense foods on the market. Their low cost, ready availability and huge benefits make them a vital part of any diet. No matter what your diet and fitness goals, fitting these superfoods into your daily diet is a great way to enjoy a healthier lifestyle, and maybe even a longer life.

In addition, the superfoods identified by science are of such a wide variety that there are sure to be superfoods to suit every taste. No matter what types of foods you favor, chances are you will be able to enjoy these great foods as part of your daily diet.

We all know how difficult it can be to make a major change to diet and lifestyle. Whether your goal is to increase your level of fitness, lose the weight you've wanted to lose, or just enjoy a healthier lifestyle and a longer life, these great foods can make that goal much easier to reach. By packing so much nutrition into such a small package, superfoods are able to provide benefits unrivaled by other foods.

Superfoods are an incredibly valuable addition to any diet, and these powerful foods, culinary herbs and supplements have proven their worth in study after study. What makes superfoods so attractive is that they are able to bring nutritional balance, and their value has long been known in the natural health and alternative medicine community.

The superfoods listed in this publication are all natural enzyme rich whole foods that are simply packed with vitamins, minerals, phytochemicals and antioxidants. From the acai berry to thyme, these foods are wholesome, easy to find, and inexpensive to buy. Even more important, the nutritional value they provide may be able to ward off some very serious diseases, including two of the biggest killers – cancer and heart disease.

The desire not only to enjoy a healthier current lifestyle but also to ward off future health problems has led to an explosion of interest in these superfoods. As the population continues to age, this interest in diet, nutrition and health is only likely to grow. Study after study has shown that diet has a significant impact on health, and often the foods we eat today will continue to impact our lives decades from now.

That is why educating yourself about the power of superfoods is such a valuable use of your time. By choosing these nutrient dense foods, herbs and supplements, you can not only feel better today, but you will be able to enjoy a healthier lifestyle and fewer health problems throughout your long life.

The benefits of a healthy diet are many, and these benefits are becoming more and more well known with every passing year. Superfoods take healthy eating to a higher level and their inclusion in a balanced diet can provide the extra boost you need to avoid cancer and heart disease, boost the effectiveness of your immune system, and even slow down the aging process.

While all the superfoods listed can provide exceptional health benefits, however, it is important to know that how such foods are harvested, processed, packaged and handled can have a significant impact on their quality, both as foods and as nutritional components.

Improper packaging can greatly affect the quality of edible, herbal and supplement varieties of superfoods. It is important to buy edible varieties of superfoods from the best supermarkets and grocery stores, and to make sure they are selected at the peak of freshness. When opting for herbal superfoods, it is generally best to select fresh herbs instead of their dried counterparts. When choosing dried herbs, however, it is important to again select them from the best stores, and to buy dried herbs that are made by the best manufacturers.

When it comes to buying superfoods as supplements, it is again important to buy only from the highest quality manufacturers. Buying supplements from the best manufacturers, those who have years of experience in the business, will help ensure that they contain only the freshest and purest ingredients, and that they have been manufactured to exacting quality standards.